Comprehensive Herbalism for Beginners Guide

(2 Books in 1)

Grow Medicinal Herbs to Fill Your Herbalist Apothecary with Natural Herbal Remedies and Plant Medicine

The Art of Herbal Healing
Content

HERB LIST

AILMENTS & REMEDIES LIST

Grow Your Own Medicine Contents

Herb List

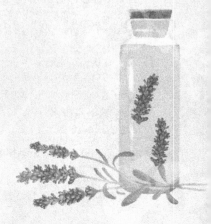

THE ART OF
HERBAL
HEALING

*Herbalism for
Beginners*

AVA GREEN

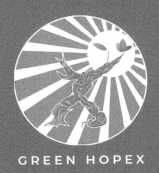

GREEN HOPEX

Content

HERB LIST

AILMENTS & REMEDIES LIST

Have questions or need advice?

JOIN our Herbal FAM JAM!

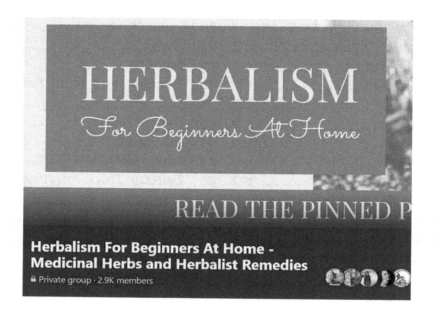

Connect with like-minded people in our private herbal community on Facebook.

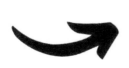

Scan with your camera to join!

www.theherb.space/group

Introduction

How much money does the average developed country spend on healthcare each year? Hundreds of billions; trillions even. The sum for most first-world countries is nearly out of the realm of our understanding and yet, most of the population struggles to stay healthy. We live on a constant adrenaline rush, heading to work, or to school. We are on the go and, while we live our busy lives, we allow toxins in. We don't have time to be selective about what goes into our bodies, and we tend to pop a pill whenever we need to forget about our discomfort. The result of this is a high level of ambivalence towards taking pills and an increased dependence on such drugs.

Undoubtedly, we need conventional Western medicine. Many serious illnesses require a drug-based approach to keep us enlivened and energized. But that doesn't mean that we should rely on it blindly. Before modern medicine, people were living their lives in a wholesome and healthy way. There were lethal diseases that medicinal plants couldn't battle, of course, but we can embrace conventional medicine in those situations. For everything else, let's find the cure in the natural world!

Over the last couple of decades, public awareness of herbal medicine has skyrocketed. People are slowly regaining trust in nature and realizing that our role intertwines with the planet's existence. We are creatures of the Earth. Handle her carefully and she will care for you in return.

Herbs are packed with active constituents that can

stimulate, support, restrain, and retrain different parts of our bodies, restoring their normal function. When used wisely, plants with therapeutic properties can work in harmony with our bodies to produce balanced health.

There are thousands of therapeutic plants, each with the ability to address and heal certain health issues. This book covers 40 of the most effective and commonly used ones, to give you a decent nudge in the right direction. Start with these herbs, and you boast hundreds of options for natural treatments in the case of most health troubles. In this book, you will also find 71 aliments and their corresponding remedies. These are merely shadows on the wall of all the wonderful uses for medicinal plants.

With 15 different extraction methods explained in detail, and bonus recipes that will help you start your healing journey right away, this will be your go-to herbal source whenever you feel like whipping up a natural cure. From how to harvest, extract, preserve, and store the herbs and their remedies, to when, and how to use them, I am sharing my ultimate secrets about the ancient art of herbal healing with every aspiring herbalist.

No fancy tools are needed, no extensive knowledge of biology required; all you need for this healing journey is the willingness to take it! Follow the advice wisely and safely, and a hale and hearty living is guaranteed

Note before reading

This book offers knowledge on how to extract medicinal herbs and make herbal remedies to address many health issues. It is a beginner-friendly guide, free of heavy and complex terminology, offering a simple and step-by-step approach to herbalism.

It is not, by any means, an herbal encyclopedia or an advanced book for well-seasoned herbalists.

The book is written by an experienced and knowledgeable herbalism enthusiast, not a physician. No parts of this book are meant to replace the advice of a medical professional. Use the herbs with caution and refer to the safety sections first. Always research the herbs well before using them, and consult with your physician for any uncertainties.

The author of this book cannot guarantee the effect of the remedies, as we all have unique conditions and requirements. The author cannot be held accountable for any injuries, misinterpretations, improper use, possible side effects or any adverse consequences.

The
Gifts of Mother Nature

When I first began to explore the benefits of herbal medicine, I started with the basics – lavender, chamomile, calendula, garlic. I had grown up watching my nana and mother do wonders with the herbs from our backyard. To me, they had seemed like magicians mixing up potions. The magic of these plants was instilled in me young. As I grew, my curiosity about the world of natural remedies expanded and I actually gave this medicine a shot when I got married. I planted my own garden. Now I have more than 30 different medicinal plants always at my fingertips, and a whole pantry stocked with remedies that help me fight diseases and keep illnesses at bay.

I was lucky enough to become familiarized with herbal healing from a very young age, so I didn't approach it with skepticism. But for those who think that the herbalism boom is nothing more than taking Instagram-worthy shots of colorful dried plants, or that herbal potions are only for big-nosed witches, allow me to show you a more accurate picture of the path to herbal healing.

Herbal healing may have been born out of necessity but even in this modern era we still walk the path paved by our ancestors. Conventional medicine may be needed in some cases, but we often forget that people in the past relied solely on what Mother Nature had to offer. And with antibiotics and other medical treatments sometimes having negative effects, therapeutic herbs are regaining the trust they lost. So many pathogens are becoming resistant to chemically loaded drugs.

As far as we know, Mother Nature has given us 50,000 to 70,000 plants with therapeutic properties; small shrubs, lichens, tiny fungi, green mosses, tall trees. It is up to us, the modern practitioners, to discover these medicinal herbs and learn how to extract their healing properties in safe and effective ways. And people have been doing that since the dawn of humanity. Every culture in the world has its own herbal traditions, whether sensible or magical, and a unique connection to nature: the oldest medicine.

Europe

Europe's herbalism history was mainly influenced by Asian practices but can be traced back to Hippocrates, an Ancient Greek philosopher, who lived from 460 −377 BC. By classifying the herbs as hot, dry, cold, or moist, Hippocrates set the foundation of traditional herbal healing. His "four humors" represented the four bodily fluids (phlegm, blood, yellow bile, and black bile) and how they corresponded with the four elements of nature (water, fire, air, and earth).

Hippocrates developed a base of healing in Greece, and herbalism quickly took over the Earth's cradle. Greece's major urban centers soon came along for the ride. Rome happily started to learn about the properties of herbal medicine. The majority of traditional knowledge of herbalism in Rome actually came from Dioscorides, who was a Roman army surgeon from AD 40−90. After observing 600 plants, he wrote his *De Materia Medica*, which further shed light on the use of plants for therapeutic purposes.

Although folk medicine was handed down from one generation to the next, European herbalism reached its apex in the 15th century, thanks to the invention of printing. In the following centuries, many herbalists managed to print herbal catalogs, in various languages, and to share their application secrets with the public. The most notable herbal reference books come from two English herbalists. John Gerard's novel *The Herbail* (1597), and Nicholas Culpeper's *The English Physitian* (1652) are the gems of herbalism in Europe. Ever since their publication, they have been providing valuable knowledge and herbal information for anyone looking to explore (or exploit) the gifts of Mother Nature.

With the rise of importation in the 17th and 18th centuries, foreign herbs were introduced into Europe. European herbalists now had the chance to expand their knowledge and improve practices. And they did so with vigor! In the 18th century, almost 70% of all medicinal plants used in Europe were imported.

When conventional medicine saw a rise in popularity, herbalism was slowly but surely cast aside. Once the pharmaceutical monopoly spread across Europe, it became illegal to practice herbalism without a special medical certificate. It was only four decades ago that herbalism started to regain its glory. Now there are many modern practitioners of herbal medicine and, in some European countries, natural remedies are routinely prescribed.

The Middle East and India

If you're into herbalism, then you've probably heard of *Ayurveda medicine.* Ayurveda is the oldest Middle Eastern and Indian healing system. It stretches way beyond simple treatment, into the realms of religion, philosophy, and science. These are considered the main components of one's being. At its core, the use of therapeutic herbs, yoga, meditation, and other practices help one reach total harmony.

This ancient practice has used medicinal plants, such as turmeric, since 4,000 BC. Early common people worked with herbal medicine for many generations, but the first official Ayurvedic school was founded in 400 BC by Punarvasu Atreya. This opened up a whole world of herbal healing for the doctors of old. Most herbs and healing minerals were discovered by the popular ancient Indian herbalists Charaka and Sushurta, in the first millennium BC.

This unique holistic approach is known to be one of the oldest medicinal practices. With Buddhism's rise, from 563–483 BC, and onward, Ayurveda became known throughout Asia, and would eventually spread to most of the developed world.

Although the British banned Ayurveda completely in the 19th century, by the time India became independent there were many herbalists ready to resurrect this healing approach. Since 1947, Ayurveda has been known as a valid and effective natural treatment system throughout the world.

China and Southeast Asia

China is the only country in the world that can brag about having an ancient herbal healing tradition that is as appreciated by people as is conventional Western medicine. Although Chinese folk medicine has been around since humans first began wandering through Asia, their traditional herbalism dates from sometime around 200 BC. The first ideas are recorded in the Chinese manuscript, *Yellow Emperor's Classic of Internal Medicine*. The main concepts throughout the book teach that life is at the mercy of the natural laws.

Traditional Chinese Medicine (TCM) has two systems: one is based on the principles of *yin* and *yang*, and the other on the five elements (wood, fire, water, earth, and metal). The principles of *yin* and *yang* state that everything has a complementary opposite; light and dark, and good and evil. The five-element system describes how our internal organs are classified and connected. The two TCM branches developed separately, and five-element healing wasn't born until sometime between the years 960–1279, during the Song dynasty.

Chinese herbalism is quite unique. Instead of just trying to cure the symptoms, a TCM practitioner seeks to find what causes the disharmony in the body. It is a much more effective approach to healing because it goes beyond symptom relief. For instance, if you catch a cold, a Chinese herbal practitioner will not just prescribe you a tincture or infusion to help you get better. He or she will observe your whole being to find out why your body hasn't adjusted well to the external factors such as wind and temperature.

Ancient Chinese medicine has greatly influenced the rest of southeast Asia, mostly Japan and Korea. The traditional Japanese medicine called *Kampoh* dates from the 5th century. This form of medicine was inspired by TCM. In Korea, herbal remedies are very similar to those used in traditional Chinese medicine.

Although TCM is now widely recognized and used for healing, it mostly addresses chronic conditions. For more serious and acute illnesses, it is replaced with conventional Western medicine, even in China.

Africa

The oldest preserved medical record in Africa is the Ebers Papyrus, which dates back to around 1550 BC. Although it is now believed to have been nothing more than a copy of previous medical collections, it clearly shows us that herbs have been used for their therapeutic properties since ancient times in Africa. This text refers to over 700 medicinal herbs and includes more than 870 different prescriptions for unique conditions.

Although most of the herbal practices were suppressed during colonial times, many traditional African healers are well-respected throughout the world today. Colonizers attempted many times to wipe out the culture of herbal practice in Africa, but today herbal remedies are widely available both in urban and rural settings. There are many remote places on the continent that have never changed their practices. Even today, African people living in far-flung rural areas, away from hospitals and conventional medical care, depend solely on their herbal remedies. They are used for chronic, simple, and serious or life-threatening conditions.

Australia and New Zealand

Aboriginal Australians settled the island continent over 60,000 years ago and possibly have the oldest and richest herbal tradition of any culture in the world. Disastrously, with the arrival of European settlers and the disruption of Aboriginal life, much of the knowledge of their healing practices vanished into a deep, forgotten well. However, bush medicine is still used in parts of Australia, and there are current efforts to record these traditions in written form. There are still many indigenous plants, like Eucalyptus, that we use and understand, thanks to Aboriginal knowledge and practices.

Similarly, after the Maori arrived in New Zealand, some 1000 years ago, they developed their own medicinal uses for some of the indigenous plants. For example, they used *Manuka* to treat skin diseases, colds, and as a sedative. Today we also know *Manuka* as a type of tea tree (*Leptospermum scoparium*), and its oil is prized as an herbal remedy. Some of our knowledge of the ways in which Maori used medicinal plants comes from the records written by the early European settlers and missionaries.

In the last 200 years, plants from Australia and New Zealand have become part of herbal medicine throughout the world. And after 1989, when the Therapeutic Goods Act (an act of Australian legislation) was passed, Australia and New Zealand started developing their herbal medicine industry, offering many natural, over-the-counter alternatives. They also commenced with commercial cultivation of therapeutic herbs, and even offer university training for aspiring practitioners.

North and Central America

The history of herbalism in North America stems from rural practices in Central America. The first American evidence of these medical cures is *The Badianus Manuscript* from 1552. It is an Aztec list of Mexican herbs used for healing purposes.

Shamanism, a religious practice that involves interacting with spirits, is closely tied to herbal healing in Central America. What is so intriguing about American herbalism is that throughout the northern and southern continents, from Canada to Chile, native people believed herbs to be bursting with spiritual energy, and packed with healing powers.

When European settlers arrived in North America, in the 17th century, they slowly realized the nature of these practices. The native people were thought to be primitive but, in fact, their herbal medicine was effective. Settlers discovered they could learn from these people and thus a knot was tied between Native American and Western herbalism. This knot inspired Dr. Wooster Beech to found Eclecticism in the 1830s, and combine herbal tradition with new scientific knowledge. By 1909, there were over 8,000 followers and practitioners of the new movement.

The practice of herbal medicine in the United States started declining in the early 20th century due to the fact that plants couldn't be patented. This meant that all pharmaceutical companies could develop herbal medicines, so competition was stiff and profits decreased. The rich and powerful threw their money behind allopathic (conventional) medical schools and the others slowly died. Practicing doctors practiced what they were taught so, once there were only allopathic schools, herbal knowledge lost favor. When supportive legislation was passed in 1994, herbalism in America let out a whoop of delight and began

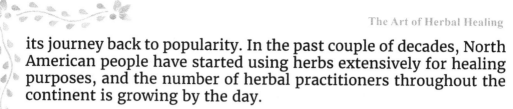
its journey back to popularity. In the past couple of decades, North American people have started using herbs extensively for healing purposes, and the number of herbal practitioners throughout the continent is growing by the day.

South America

When thinking of South American herbalism, the first things that come to mind are rituals, sacrifices, and magic. South America is known to have many hallucinogenic plants that allowed its native people to "communicate" with spirits. But beyond shamanism, there is a wide variety of different herbal practices and traditions throughout the continent. From the Amazon region to the city of Rio de Janeiro, each South American culture is dominated by specific plants and their usages. Thanks to the abundance of thick rainforests, South America holds the title of the continent with the most mysterious, unexplained, and unexplored medicinal potential.

With the Spanish conquests in the 16th century, Europeans started exporting plants to Europe. Soon after this, native South American herbal traditions and secret remedies spread throughout the world. Today, in South America, herbal practitioners combine native and Western methods of healing.

Tragically, South American herbalism, and many of the native medicinal plants, are under threat of becoming extinct as, every year, more of the rainforests are cut down or further exploited by money-hungry corporations.

Irrespective of herbalism's history, today there is a growing interest in medicinal plants throughout the world. As the non-selective use of conventional drugs is on the rise, the effects that these drugs have on diseases has started to decrease. This forces us to look for alternative treatments to complement the conventional drugs, so that we can have these drugs as a reserve to use only when necessary. And herbalism offers just that. Read on to see exactly how you can benefit from this natural approach to healing.

Learning the Ropes

You may be tempted to skip this chapter and get straight to the nitty-gritty of using herbs for medicinal purposes, but I strongly suggest otherwise. Before you reach for your mortar and pestle, and grab a handful of your windowsill herbs, you first need to make sure that you know the basis of herbalism. One must develop a strong foundation to moderate one's expectations and returns.

The Benefits of Herbalism

Herbalism involves the use of plants with therapeutic properties, from which the biological compounds are extracted and then used to treat various physical and mental health conditions. Herbal medicine is not some cryptic science without proven treatment methods. The World Health Organization (WHO) has estimated that approximately 80% of the overall population depends on natural medicine for some form of health care.

Apart from the obvious benefit of addressing health issues, there are many other reasons you should give herbalism a try:

Economic Benefits – One of the main reasons herbal medicine is so popular is because medicinal plants are quite cost-effective. You can summon up a large batch of remedies with just a few tablespoons of a single herb.

Sense of Self-Reliance – Knowing how to whip up your own natural medicaments means you are no longer dependent on the pharmaceutical industry for alleviating every physical discomfort. There is a rewarding aspect to creating your own balms and potions. Whenever I take a glimpse at my well-stocked home apothecary, I feel a pleasant sense of accomplishment.

Safe and Natural Alternative – Creating your own herbal medicine means there is no guesswork involved, no wondering what is inside your remedy bottles. There are no hidden ingredients, and no harmful chemicals added. Think of it as squeezing nature's goodness straight into your jars.

Healthier Alternative – Herbal remedies really pack a punch! Unlike conventional medicine which is produced with the sole purpose of treating symptoms, medicinal plants go beyond addressing a certain health issue. Take rosemary, for instance. Rosemary infusion can act as a powerful remedy for treating migraines, but that's not the only thing it does. Rosemary is a decent source of vitamins A, B_6, and C, as well as the minerals calcium and iron. These medicaments are not only treating the ailment but giving you other benefits as well. This sure beats a chemical painkiller, doesn't it?

It Gives You Options – Herbs have different medicinal uses (more on those in the next section) that stimulate our cells. The best thing about making your homemade remedies is the ability to mix and match! You can combine herbs as you see fit, to address your unique conditions, and adjust their intensities in a way that works for your health. The possibilities are quite endless.

The Anatomy of Herbs

It is easy to find out what medicinal effects a certain herb has on the body. Simple research can tell you which herbs you need to take for inflammation, calming your nerves, or alleviating pain. And that should work fine for a one-time remedy. But if you are serious about trying your hand at herbalism and creating plant-based medicaments, then you need a much deeper approach.

Apart from knowing the medicinal effects, you also need to understand the anatomy of herbs; different parts of the plants produce different compounds, all of which have certain actions within the body. Knowing a bit about the herbs' active constituents and their chemical compositions will help you understand how they work, which will kickstart your journey to becoming a master herbal healer.

Volatile Oils – Volatile oil is the plant's extract that we use for making essential oil. Usually composed of more than 100 different compounds, mostly monoterpenes (molecules with ten carbon atoms), it is one of the most important herbal constituents for medicinal purposes.

Phenols – Phenols are herbal constituents that are mainly antiseptic or anti-inflammatory in nature. They are usually produced by plants as a defense mechanism to protect themselves against external infection or grazing by insects. Some phenolic acids are powerful antioxidants and can even be antiviral. Phenols are a very varied group of organic compounds, but each compound is highly effective.

Tannins – Almost all plants produce tannins. Once again, this active constituent has the power to repel herbivorous insects. Tannin is a polyphenolic compound and a powerful astringent. In herbal medicine, this compound is mostly used for its ability to promote blood clotting and staunch bleeding. It also tightens relaxed tissues and is an effective cure for diarrhea and skin issues, such as eczema.

Flavonoids – Just like tannins, flavonoids are polyphenolic compounds that can be found in most plants. Flavonoids act as pigments, meaning they impart color (usually white or yellow) to fruits and flowers. This active constituent has many different medicinal effects, but the main reason we want to extract flavonoids is because of their powerful antioxidant uses. Plants that contain flavonoids are perfect for improving circulation, but they can also be used as anti-inflammatories, antivirals, and to protect the liver.

Coumarins – These active constituents can have quite different medicinal actions. Some plants containing coumarins stimulate the skin, while others can be powerful blood thinners and even muscle relaxants.

Saponins – If this word first reminds you of the word 'soap', you are not far from the truth. This active compound is called *saponin* because it makes a lather when it comes into contact with water, just like soap. Saponins can be expectorants (promote the secretion of mucus) and help with nutrient absorption, when in their *triterpenoid* form. When they occur in a *steroidal* form, these constituents have a powerful hormonal action.

Alkaloids – Pharmacologically speaking, alkaloids are active constituents due to their nitrogen–loaded chemical composition. Alkaloid plants help to create many popular conventional drugs, but they can have a powerful effect on the body, even in their raw, natural form. Alkaloid herbs can alleviate pain, reduce muscle spasms, and even help dry up secretions.

Polysaccharides – As the name suggests, polysaccharides contain sugar molecules. This constituent is found in all plants, but the most medicinally important ones are those that resemble a sticky gum, usually found in roots, bark, leaves, and seeds. These "gums" can soak up fluids, making them perfect for soothing and repairing irritated tissues or mucous membranes. Some polysaccharides also improve the immune system, for example, the sugar molecules found in aloe vera leaves.

Bitters – As you've already guessed, bitters are the active compounds in herbs that have a bitter or harsh taste. In theory, bitterness stimulates secretions in the digestive organs, so understandably, bitter medicinal plants can be perfect for improving and soothing digestive function. Bitters also allow the body to absorb nutrients more efficiently.

Proanthocyanins – Like flavonoids and tannins, proanthocyanins are also pigments, but these compounds give a darker hint of color – think blue, red, or purple flowers. This constituent is perfect for improving circulation in the heart, but also in the eyes, hands, and feet.

Cyanogenic Glycosides – As scary as the name sounds, cyanogenic glycosides can be quite helpful in tiny doses, despite producing toxic hydrogen cyanide when the plant is crushed. They act as a powerful relaxant that sedates the heart and muscles. In fact, the leaves, stems, seeds and roots of the elder tree contain these active substances, which is why their use can have a soothing effect.

Cardiac Glycosides – As the name suggests, these herbal

constituents can protect the heart and entire cardiovascular system. They support the contraction rate and impact positively on the heart's function. But cardiac glycosides can also act as a diuretic and are incredibly helpful for urine production as well. Foxgloves are one of the best sources of these active compounds.

Anthraquinones – These herbal compounds do wonders for the large intestine. By causing contractions and stimulating the intestine walls, anthraquinones induce bowel movement and are a perfect natural laxative for treating irritating constipation.

Glucosilinates – This active constituent is only found in plants belonging to the cabbage and mustard family, and is often quite irritating for the skin, even causing blistering. However, when applied to joints as a poultice, these compounds can increase the blood flow and support healing.

Minerals – Just like all plants, medicinal herbs are packed with minerals. Many plants draw these beneficial compounds from the ground and then convert them into something easily broken down and absorbed by the body. For instance, dandelion leaves contain a high level of potassium, in addition to being a very powerful diuretic.

Vitamins – Although this is probably the most overlooked use for medicinal plants, many herbs have considerable vitamin content. In addition to their other therapeutic actions, herbs contain vitamins that increase their ability to heal your body. The more vitamins your body gets, the better your health will be.

Speaking the Herbal Language

Before we get down to gathering herbs and extracting the active goodies trapped inside, it is beneficial to go through common terminology. Knowing the essential vocabulary and herbalism concepts will prepare you better to start this therapeutic practice on the right foot.

Whether we are discussing herbal actions, preparations, plant parts, or just common terms, this full herbal glossary is one that every aspiring herbalist should be familiar with:

Abortifacient – An action that induces abortion.

Acetract/Acetum – An herbal remedy that uses vinegar to extract the active compounds from herbs.

Adaptogen – Herbs that support the adrenal glands and help us adapt to and modulate physical and emotional stress.

Adjuvant – An agent which supports the actions of medicinal agents.

Alterative – An action that helps with chronic conditions because it removes metabolic wastes, boosts immunity, and cleanses the body.

Amoebicidal – Herbs that help with diseases caused by an amoeba.

Amphoteric – Actions that restore the normal functioning of organs.

Anabolic – Meaning to promote healthy tissue growth.

Analeptic – To stimulate and restore the normal functioning of the central nervous system.

Analgesic – An herbal action that relieves pain.

Anaphrodisiac – An action that is the opposite of aphrodisiac, meaning it reduces sexual desire and arousal.

Anesthetic – An action that induces anesthesia, numbness or loss of sensation by depressing certain nerve functions   .

Antacid – An agent which neutralizes stomach acidity.

Anti-anemic – A medium which prevents anemia or helps with treating it, if already present.

Antibacterial – Prevents bacteria from spreading.

Antibilious – An action that combats stomachache, nausea, and other conditions that are caused by increased bile secretions.

Antibiotic – An action that inhibits bacterial growth.

Anticancerous – Prevents or decreases the risk of developing cancer.

Anticatarrh – Herbs that help with inflamed mucous membranes of throat and head.

Antidepressant – Medicinal action that prevents or decreases the intensity of mental depression.

Antidiabetic – An agent that helps with diabetes and may even improve the utilization of insulin.

Antidiarrheal (antidiarrhetic) – An action that prevents or treats diarrhea.

Anti-emetic – Alleviates and even prevents vomiting and nausea.

Anti-epileptic – An action that relieves symptoms of epilepsy and combats seizures.

Antifungal – An instrument used to destroy the growth of fungi.

Antihemorrhagic – Alleviates hemorrhaging and controls or prevents bleeding.

Anti-infectious – Stops or prevents infections.

Anti-inflammatory – An action that controls, reduces and prevents inflammation in the body.

Antilithic – Prevents kidney or bladder stones from forming.

Antimalarial – Relieves patient from symptoms or prevents malaria.

Antimicrobial – Herbs that destroy microbes.

Antioxidant – Prevents oxidation.

Antiparasitic – An action that prevents parasites from building up or treats parasitic conditions, if already present.

Antiperiodic – Herbal action that prevents diseases (like malaria) from reoccurring periodically.

Antiphlogistic – An action that counteracts inflammation.

Antipruritic – Prevents and relieves aggravating symptoms of itching.

Antipyretic – Reduces body fever and induces perspiration.

Antirheumatic – Prevents, treats, and eases the pain caused by rheumatism, an inflammation of the muscles and joints.

Antiscorbutic – Prevents and treats scurvy, a disease caused by vitamin C deficiency.

Antiseptic – An action that prevents decay, removes blood and pus, and inhibits the development of microorganisms.

Antispasmodic – Calms the nervous system and prevents and relieves muscle cramp and spasm.

Antitussive – Prevents, controls, and relieves coughing.

Anti-ulcer – Prevents ulcers from forming.

Antivenomous – An action that can act as a prevention to animal poison.

Antiviral – Works against viruses.

Antizymotic – An agent that prevents fermentation or decomposition.

Anxiolytic – Herbal action that prevents, relieves and reduces symptoms of anxiety.

Aperient – Works as a gentle laxative.

Aperitive – Herbs that are taken before meals to stimulate and increase appetite.

Aphrodisiac – Restores and increases sexual desire and arousal.

Aromatherapy – The art and practice of using essential oils to promote physical and emotional health. Aromatherapy stimulates the receptor sites in the brain, allowing the compounds from the oils to be absorbed.

Aromatic – Herbs that are rich in volatile oils and fragrant compounds.

Asepsis – Sterile and uninfected; free of germs.

Astringent – An action that causes the skin, blood vessels, and tissues to contract. It stops bleeding and mucus discharge.

Aquaretic – Increases urine production while retaining electrolytes. Great for improving blood circulation in the kidneys, but without affecting sodium resorption.

Bactericidal – Herbs that prevent bacterial infections.

Balsam – Soothing tree resin.

Bronchial – Improves respiration by relaxing spasms in the lungs and/or the tubes leading to them.

Calmative – Soothing actions with sedative properties.

Carcinostatic – Halting the growth of malignant tumors and carcinomas.

Cardiotonic – An action that strengthens the functioning of the heart.

Carminative – Prevents the formation of gas in the intestines and helps its release.

Cathartic – Induces bowel movement and causes evacuation. Cathartic herbs can be mild or vigorous.

Caustic – Herbs that are rich in acid that can cause corrosion on living tissues.

Cephalic – A term that refers to diseases on, in or near the head.

Cholagogue – An action that improves the flow of bile in the gallbladder.

Cicatrizant – Improves wound healing and supports the recovery of scar tissue.

Cordial – A stimulating herbal drink or medicine.

Counterirritant – An action that causes an inflammatory response of the affected area.

Decongestant – Relieves congestion.

Demulcent – Soothes, relieves, and protects irritated or inflamed mucous membrane, both internally and externally.

Deobstruent – Clears duct obstruction for the normal flow of secretions and bodily fluids.

Depurative – An action that purifies and cleanses the blood.

Dermatitis – Skin inflammation that results in itchiness and redness, also known as rash.

Detergent – Cleanses wounds, infections, ulcers, and boils.

Diaphoretic – An action that promotes perspiration and circulation, and eliminates surface toxins.

Digestive – Supports and promotes healthy digestion.

Disinfectant – Herbal action that destroys germs and pathogenic microbes that cause infections.

Diuretic – Herbal action that promotes the production and flow of urine.

Ecbolic – Increases uterine contractions.

Emetic – Herbs that induce and cause vomiting and the emptying of stomach contents.

Emmenagogue – Supports and regulates normal menstrual flow, but it can also clear blood congestion.

Emollient – Actions that soothe and soften the skin.

Epispastic – Substances that cause a discharge or blister to form.

Errhine – Herbal action that increases nasal secretion, as well as stimulating sneezing, when applied to the mucus membrane.

Escharotic – A substance that causes sloughing and kills tissue.

Estrogenic – An action that increases the production of the hormone estrogen, or acts as an estrogen.

Euphoriant – Sometimes addictive, this medicinal action causes the body to enter a temporary euphoric state.

Exanthematous – A remedy for measles, scarlet fever, and similar eruptive diseases of the skin.

Exhilarant – An herbal action that uplifts the mood and cheers the mind.

Expectorant – Supports the removal of the mucus from the trachea and lungs, although this term is often used to explain all sorts of remedies that can relieve coughs.

Febrifuge – An action that can decrease body temperature and fever. Very similar to antipyretic.

Galactagogue – Increases and supports the production and healthy flow of breast milk.

Germicide – An action that can destroy germs (pathogens).

Hemagogue – Supports and promotes healthy blood flow.

Hemostatic – Herbs that are astringent and can staunch or control bleeding, and purify the blood.

Hepatic – Increases bile secretion and promotes healthy liver function.

Hypertensive – An action that increases blood pressure.

Hypnotic – Relaxes the nervous system and supports sleep.

Hypoglycemiant – An action that lowers the blood sugar level.

Hypotensive – An action that lowers the blood pressure.

Inhalation – Breathing in steam through the nasal passage.

Laxative – Promotes the evacuation of bowel contents.

Lithotriptic – Substances that cause kidney and bladder stones to dissolve.

Liniment – An external remedy that is applied by rubbing.

Masticatory – Substances that increase the production of saliva when chewing.

Mucilage/Mucilaginous – A sticky substance secreted by mucous membranes and glands.

Mydriatic (also Myotic) – An action that causes the pupils to dilate.

Narcotic – Addictive substance that reduces pain and induces drowsiness or sleep.

Nauseant – Causes vomiting and nausea.

Nervine – An action that relaxes the nervous system, soothes the nerves, and decreases tension.

Nootropic – Substances that improve cognitive functions and improve concentration and memory.

Oxytocic – An action that induces uterine contractions.

Parasiticide – Herbs that can destroy parasites.

Parturifacient – Induces labor and childbirth.

Refrigerant – Cooling actions that get rid of thirst and/or remove heat.

Relaxant – Substances that relax and get rid of anxiety and tension.

Renal – An action that strengthens, supports and treats kidney diseases and imbalances.

Rubefacient – Increases skin blood flow and induces redness.

Sedative – Substances that promote sleep and bring tranquility.

Soporific – Similar to a sedative. It promotes sleep.

Spasmodic – Causes muscle contraction and relaxation.

Steroids – Active organic compounds that include alkaloids, some vitamins and some hormones.

Stimulant – Stimulates and increases the functioning of a certain body part or organ, temporarily.

Stomachic – Promotes the health of the stomach and supports normal digestion.

Terpenes – Hydrocarbon molecules that are aromatic and form the base of volatile oils.

Tonic – Herbs that strengthen, restore, and nourish the entire body.

Topical – Form of remedy application that is used externally, on the body's surface.

Thymoleptic – Modifies mood and energizes mental health and wellbeing.

Vermicide/Vermifuge – Substance that destroys intestinal worms.

Vulnerary – Supports wound healing.

Now that you know how medicinal plants work and why you should give herbalism a try, the real fun can begin. Let's dive deeper into the therapeutic side of nature, so that we can learn how to allow it to heal us from the inside out.

The Most Effective Herbs to Know, Grow and Use

erbs are the cornerstone of healing, and they have been used for medicinal practices for thousands of years. They may be masked by various chemical processes, but plant compounds still form the foundation of many pharmaceuticals that we use today. Did you know that aspirin is derived from willow bark? No, I am not railing against the use of modern drugs; I am simply trying to emphasize the potency that natural herbs have. When your body starts to shoot off painful signals, it is tempting to reach for that bottle of pills – but there is an alternative!

Herbs comprise many active components, each bringing something new and different to the body. They produce various chemical compounds that can protect against, or help treat, many diseases and illnesses. Depending on what health concerns you are looking to address, there are many herbs, or parts of plants, that you can use to your advantage.

To break free from the unnecessary shackles of the pharmaceutical industry, I present to you the 40 essential herbs that will help you build your natural apothecary at home.

Your Natural First-Aid Kit

We all have a first-aid kit somewhere around the house, in the trunk of our car, or stashed somewhere else; while this conventional suitcase is well-equipped to assist us when we are in an accident, that doesn't mean that we should reach for chemically-loaded creams for every scrape. Enriching the medical bag with natural supplements not only gives you more options to choose from when a sudden injury strikes, but also helps you limit the use of pharmaceuticals when it is not necessary.

To make sure you are shielded from all sorts of misfortunes, here are the top 12 herbs that every green healer wannabe should never run out of.

ARNICA
(Arnica montana)

Arnica montana is a powerful homeopathic that is mostly used for relieving muscle pain. A 2007 study found that arnica gel was just as effective as Ibuprofen gel when given to patients with finger osteoarthritis (Widrig et al., 2007). Both groups had a similar recovery, and the doctors had a difficult time distinguishing between those patients who received the arnica, and those who received the Ibuprofen gel.

My husband often has claudication (leg cramps when walking) so, whenever we take our long walks or go hiking, I always have my arnica gel with me. I remember once he started experiencing severe calf pain, and he could barely move. We sat on the ground, and I massaged this amazing gel into the skin on his leg for about ten minutes or so. Half an hour later, he was ready to race me to the top of the hill.

Native to: Europe, Northwestern US, Canada, the Pyrenees Mountains, Siberia

Description: When harvested in full bloom, arnica is recognizable by its yellow flowers and egg-shaped leaves. Arnica is mostly used as a natural ointment and compression for sprains and bruises. It kickstarts the healing process and relieves muscle pain. It can be used, internally, for treating shock or injury, but this is a rare application and requires dilution. The plant can be quite toxic (even if the dose is low), so internal consumption is not recommended.

Arnica cream or gel can be the perfect addition to your natural first-aid kit and effective for healing bruises or decreasing muscl aches.

Main Components: Flavonoids, sesquiterpene lactones, volatil oil, polysaccharides, mucilage, thymol

Medicinal Actions:
Homeopathic
Anti-inflammatory

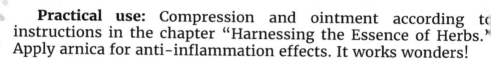

Main Uses:
Relieves Muscle Pain
Heals Bruises and Sprains
Improves Blood Supply Locally
Reabsorbs Internal Bleeding

Parts Used: The flowers and rhizome

Practical use: Compression and ointment according to instructions in the chapter "Harnessing the Essence of Herbs." Apply arnica for anti-inflammation effects. It works wonders!

Safety Precautions: Arnica, in its pure form, can be quite poisonous when taken internally. Use only for external application and only when the skin is healthy. Applying arnica on broken skin can cause dermatitis.

CALENDULA
(Calendula officinalis)

Calendula tinctures are probably the most effective natural tissue-repairing and redness-soothing remedy. Its pharmacological properties and high anti-inflammatory constituents make calendula the safest wash for infants' diaper rash.

I always keep a calendula ointment in my first-aid kit bag, as it always comes in handy in late spring, when the sun gets a bit too hot for my skin. The herb also makes fantastic natural gargles for sore throats and blisters. A few years back, when I was going through a tough period, doctors diagnosed that stress was causing painful blisters in my mouth. If it hadn't been for my calendula gargles to relieve these sores, I would probably have been even more stressed.

Native to: Southern Europe

Description: You may know it as pot marigold, that lovely orange flower sitting decoratively in your garden. But what you may not be aware of is that calendula is packed with medicinal properties that should grant it a place in your first-aid kit. Primarily used as a remedy for the skin, calendula can soothe inflamed skin, rashes, and sunburns, and is also effective for cuts and scrapes. When taken internally, these bright orange petals support digestion and help against gut inflammation issues.

Main Components: Flavonoids, resins, phytosterols, carotenes, bitter glycosides, mucilage, volatile oil.

Medicinal Actions:
Anti-inflammatory
Antiviral
Antibacterial
Detoxifying
Heals Wounds
Relieves Muscle Spasms
Mildly Estrogenic

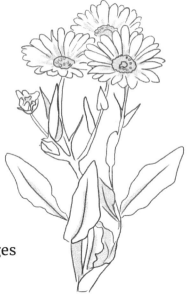

Main Uses:
Soothes Red and Inflamed Skin (rashes, burns, acne)
Treats Fungal Conditions (thrush, athlete's foot, ringworm)
Treats *Candida albicans* Efficiently
Heals Cuts and Wounds (it astringes the capillaries)
Supports Digestion
Helps with Ulcers and Gastritis
Gynecological Uses

Parts Used: The flowers: the petals and the flower head

Practical use: Suitable for making infusions, infused oils, creams, ointments, and tinctures.

Safety Precautions: Don't take calendula internally during pregnancy. It can also cause drowsiness if combined with post-surgery medications, and chronic sleepiness if consumed with sedatives.

COMFREY
(Symphytum officinale)

Comfrey is one of the most powerful natural healers. My homemade ointment is always in my medical kit to assist with sprains and bruises. Accompanying my husband on his hiking adventures goes against my clumsy nature, as I always seem to find a huge rock on which to sprain my ankle. My record was last fall when my clumsiness clashed with rainy weather and a slippery path. I seemed always to be injuring myself. Multiple times on the trail, I twisted my ankle. I thought my husband would have to carry me all the way back but, after 20 minutes of rubbing the ointment on my injury, I was actually able to get up and walk normally. Comfrey may not be magical, but it sure is effective.

Don't just blindly believe me. Research from the Complementary Therapies in Medicine *(Frost et al., 2013) suggests that comfrey is quite effective in healing abrasive wounds.*

Native to: Europe

Description: If you live in a temperate region, you have probably come across comfrey before. With thick leaves and a cluster of (usually) pink flowers, this shrub grows throughout the world. Comfrey, literally meaning *made firm*, has a long history of traditional use for mending bones. In fact, the common names for comfrey are knitbone and boneset, because of this classic application. It can also be used for healing wounds and ruptures. Today, this beneficial plant is a popular natural supplement used to treat sports injuries, thanks to its powerful ability to support the healing of bruises, fractures, and sprains. Comfrey can also be used for treating insect bites or other skin-inflammation issues.

Main Components: Mucilage, phenolic acids, allantoin, asparagine, triterpenoids, tannins

Medicinal Actions:
Anti-inflammatory
Demulcent
Tissue-repairing Properties

Wound-healing Actions
Astringent

Main Uses:
Supports the Healing of Bruises
Knits Together Ligaments and Bones
Reduces the Severity of Sprains as Compress
Applied for Graze Soothing
Heals Insects Bites
Used for Treating Mastitis

Parts Used: Entire plant – roots and aerial parts

Practical use: Feel free to make a compress, tincture, ointment or infused oil out of comfrey, for the desired outcome.

Safety Precautions: Comfrey can be unsafe for internal use as it has been linked to liver damage. For this reason, it has become a much-maligned plant. It is certainly one herb that should be used under the guidance of a practitioner until you have sufficient experience of your own. It is very valuable for use internally, and in the short term, once you know how to use it. When applying externally, make sure that the skin is healthy and not broken, as the chemicals in comfrey can cause further damage.

ECHINACEA
(Echinacea spp.)

Scientists have concluded that consuming echinacea might knock down the risk of catching a cold by 58% (Shah et al.,2007). If you are already fighting a cold, the same scientists found out that taking echinacea can shorten the time you spend in bed by 1.4 days.

Last winter, I was on a weekend trip to the Alps, and the whole family got a cold in the middle of our ski trip. We had paid for everything in advance and were really looking forward to having some fun. You could only imagine how annoyed we were about having to spend the rest of our trip in bed. Since I'd brought my herbal kit along, I thought it would be a good idea for us to take an echinacea pill before going to bed. And boy, was I right. The next day, our cold symptoms were almost gone, and we had a memorable time out in the snow.

Native to: Central USA

Description: Previously referred to as *snakeroot*, echinacea is a purple daisy-like perennial packed with infection-fighting and toxin-cleansing properties. Traditionally used as a cure for snake bites, sore throat, and septic issues, this coneflower can be a powerful natural remedy for viral and bacterial conditions. Although echinacea's medicinal history is not a very long list, today, snakeroot is one of the most commonly used plants in Western herbal medicine. Echinacea can be used for various diseases, especially those related to infection.

Main Components: Polysaccharides, caffeic acid esters, alkylamines

Medicinal Actions:
Detoxifying
Anti-inflammatory
Wound Healing Properties
Antimicrobial
Immune Modulating
Increases White Blood Cell Count

Main Uses:
Remedy for Infections
Relieves Sore Throats
Relieves Acne and Other Skin Infections
Treats Asthma and Similar Allergies
Flu and Cold Remedy
Relieves Skin from Bites and Stings

Parts Used: The flower and root

Practical use: Echinacea is awesome as a tincture, when made nto capsules or tablets, or a decoction.

Safety Precautions: Echinacea is generally safe for both nternal and external use. However, keep in mind that echinacea nteracts with caffeine. Taking echinacea with coffee will slow .he breakdown of caffeine, and you may end up with too much :affeine in the bloodstream.

FEVERFEW
(Tanacetum parthenium)

Research says that feverfew has the potential to be considered :he natural drug for treating migraines (Pittler & Ernst, 2004). [t reduces the frequency and severity of migraines but is not for aspirin-like pain relief of other types of headaches. It has anti-nflammatory properties and is believed to increase the release of serotonin and decrease the release of histamines. Instead of reaching for a painkiller, why not try to soothe the ache the herbal way. The extract of this herb, in the form of capsules, is my go-to for reducing the severity of migraines.

A few months back, I was headed to a conference in another :ountry, with my husband. I always have a mean headache after a long drive, and this time was no different. Just as I thought that I would spend the whole day in agony, I popped one of my feverfew capsules, and 2 hours later, the symptoms of my migraine were gone. Surprisingly enough, my head didn't hurt on our trip back home either.

Native to: Southeastern Europe

Description: At first glance, you might confuse this plant with chamomile. Despite both belonging to the Chrysanthemum family, and sharing the same white, daisy-like flower with a yellow center, these two plants are different. Unlike chamomile, it is the leaves of the feverfew that are packed with therapeutic properties. Traditionally referred to as "the woman's herb," feverfew has been used for inducing menstruation for many centuries. Now mainly used for treating migraines, feverfew is a must-have among your herbal supplements. Keep it in your first-aid kit for quick relief.

Main Components: Volatile oil, sesquiterpenes, sesquiterpene lactones

Medicinal Actions:
Analgesic
Anti-inflammatory
Antirheumatic
Supports the Menstrual Cycle
Reduces Fevers

Main Uses:
Lowers Body Temperature
Induces Menstruation
Prevents Migraine
Decreases Arthritic and Rheumatic Pain

Parts Used: The aerial parts (the parts that grow above ground)

Practical use: Go right ahead and make a tincture, capsules or tablets, or just use the fresh leaves for consumption. So easy! It can't get any better than that!

Safety Precautions: Avoid chewing fresh leaves and internal consumption during pregnancy. Feverfew is also known to impair blood clotting, so avoid using before and after surgery.

GARLIC
(Allium sativum)

Garlic can be a powerful antibiotic, which is great for treating infections. Scientists have found that, under certain circumstances, its compound diallyl sulfide is a whopping 100 times more effective than other conventional antibiotics used for slaying the Campylobacter bacterium, the main culprit for gut infections (Lu et al., 2012). You may not be a big fan of your garlic breath, but your health will surely appreciate your consumption of the plant.

When visiting Chicago last year, my daughter started experiencing terrible pain in her ear. She always has trouble with the nerves around the ear canals when the temperature drops and she doesn't have her hat on. Just as she started to complain, I gave her a garlic capsule (an extract I always keep in my first-aid kit). After 30 to 40 minutes, when I asked her if she was feeling better, she smiled, surprised, and said, "Oh, I already forgot about the pain. I guess your magical pills do work!"

Native to: Central Asia

Description: If your grandma used to chew on garlic cloves to knock down her blood pressure, you already know of the amazing benefits of this pungent bulbous perennial. Garlic does not only enhance our meals, but it also improves our health. It fights infections, keeps our blood pressure, cholesterol, and blood sugar in check, and it is one of the most popular natural supplements. Experts say the best way to squeeze out the healthy antimicrobial compounds from garlic is to crush, dice or otherwise break the cloves to allow conversion of chemicals to allicin, and other antibiotic goodies, before tincturing or eating. Wait 10 minutes after crushing, and then use this as a medicine or ingest with food. Garlic's well-known odor comes from the sulfur compounds that it contains.

Garlic extract, in the form of capsules, can be the perfect addition to your first-aid bag to take care of sudden infections.

Main Components: Volatile oil, selenium, scordinin, vitamin A, B, C, E, allicin

Medicinal Actions:
Antibiotic
Antidiabetic
Anti-inflammatory
Expectorant
Blood Pressure Regulator
Sweat Inducer

Main Uses:
Lowers High Blood Pressure
Aid for Type 2 Diabetes
Treats Infections (mostly for the throat, nose, chest, ears)
Prevents and Breaks Down Blood Clots
Helps Treat Fungal Skin Conditions
Protects from Cancers, Such as Stomach and Colon Cancers

Parts Used: The whole plant (mostly the bulb)

Practical use: Suitable for raw consumption, syrups, capsules or tablets. All work wonderfully, depending on your needs.

Safety Precautions: Garlic is known to lower blood sugar and blood pressure, so use with caution if you already have low blood pressure or sugar, as the levels may drop too low for you. Also, raw garlic, applied to the skin, may cause irritations in some cases.

LAVENDER
(Lavandula spp.)

In the 17th century, the herbalist John Parkinson wrote about lavender, saying it was "good for the griefs and pains of the head and brain." I'm here in the 21st century to confirm what Parkinson said. A 2014 study found that consuming lavender essential oil treated anxiety more effectively than a tranquilizer (Chevallier, 2016, p. 108). But this lovely-scented herb is more than just a relaxant. Its essential oil is great for treating insect bites and burns, making it a great addition to a natural first-aid kit.

A couple of years back, we went camping with some friends. I went with my daughter a day earlier, and my husband was supposed to join us the next day. I had forgotten my herbal kit, so I asked him to bring it along. The first night we endured so many mosquito bites that we spent the next day scratching our skin off. Once he brought my lavender oil, we applied it onto the affected areas, and the irritation started to wear off. My husband also treated his own skin as a preventative measure. Take a guess as to how many mosquito bites he endured that evening . . . None!

Native to: Western Mediterranean, especially France

Description: Lavender can do more than just soothe you during a relaxing soak in the bath. You may primarily know it to be a scent in your cosmetic products or room fresheners, but lavender has powerful medicinal properties as well. When used internally, the purple flowers can be a great antidepressant, while external applications work as an insecticide. And thanks to the high content of volatile oil, lavender will also keep the health of your gut in check.

Lavender essential oil has proven to be an invaluable remedy that can even relieve headaches, if gently massaged on the temples.

Main Components: Volatile oil, flavonoids

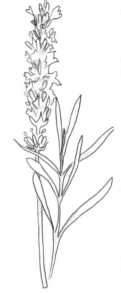

Medicinal Actions:
Antidepressant
Antispasmodic
Neuroprotective
Antimicrobial

Main Uses:
Relaxant for Reducing Stress and Anxiety
Sedative Effect
Soothes Indigestion
Soothes Insect Bites
Antiseptic for Burns, Wounds and Sores

Parts Used: The flowers

Practical use: You can make a great cup of tea just before sleep, an essential oil, tincture, infusion or even a relaxing massage oil, out of this almost magical herb.

Safety Precautions: When applying the essential oil topically, make sure to use small, medicinal amounts, as lavender can sometimes cause irritation if the dosage is higher. Also, avoid taking lavender with sedatives, as it might cause chronic sleepiness. Lavender oil is also estrogenic, so avoid using large amounts over long periods of time; for this reason, lavender oil can cause problems for children, especially small boys.

MYRRH
(Commiphora molmol)

Known as "the Wise Man's Cure," myrrh was one of the gifts that baby Jesus received from the Three Wise Men. Known as one of the oldest medicinal herbs, ancient Egyptians depended on this beneficial tree for treating herpes and hay fever. Today, studies have found that myrrh helps with neuropathic pain and rheumatoid arthritis (Chevallier, 2016, p. 85), and is a key weapon against many infections. In fact, it is one of the most powerful weapons we will discuss. One study found that myrrh extract clears liver fluke infections in a matter of weeks (Massoud et al.,

2001).

And I can attest to that! Three years ago, I started experiencing severe diarrhea and abdominal pain. I went to my doctor, and he told me it was caused by liver fluke. I researched and found out that myrrh – my sore-throat remedy – was perfect for it. In a couple of days, I wasn't feeling any more symptoms. A week after that, on my next checkup, my doctor was surprised at how I had cleansed myself with nothing but herbs. Like a green doctor in the forest, you too can mix up your own powders and potions to become more powerful.

Native to: Northeast Africa

Description: You may know myrrh as the distinct scent used in conventional mouthwashes, but in its natural state, this gummy resin oozes out of the cuts of the myrrh tree's bark. When dried, myrrh turns yellow-red, resembling raisins. Packed with anti-inflammatory properties, and having a rich, bitter taste, this gum is quite beneficial for relieving coughs, asthma, and sore throats, which is why it deserves a spot in your first-aid kit.

Main Components: Gum, volatile oil, resin

Medicinal Actions:
Anti-inflammatory
Anticancerous
Antiseptic
Antiparasitic
Anti-ulcer
Astringent

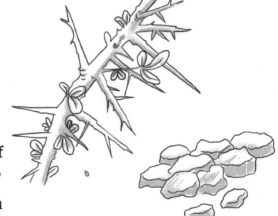

Main Uses:
Clears the Body of Parasitic Infections, Especially Liver Fluke
A Remedy for the Mouth and Throat
Ayurvedic Remedy and Tonic
Cures Ulcers
Relieves Congestion
Clears Oral Thrush
Treats Acne and other Skin Problems

Parts Used: The gum (resin)

Practical use: Myrrh can be used in tinctures, mouthwashes, powders, capsules and essential oils.

Safety Precautions: Follow the instructions for the dosage well, before consuming, as large doses of myrrh can cause kidney irritation and changes in the heart rate. Also, myrrh interacts with blood sugar medications, so avoid using this herb if you are already taking drugs for diabetes.

TEA TREE
(Melaleuca alternifolia)

It was Captain James Cook who introduced this Aboriginal remedy to the Western world in the 1770s. He had sipped a tea made from the leaves of this species of tea tree, to prevent scurvy, and asked the Aborigines (indigenous Australian people) to share its healing secrets with him. When he brought tea tree oil back to the west for the doctors to test its powers, it was confirmed that tea tree oil was a better antiseptic than the then popular aloe vera. Tea tree oil was extensively used before the discovery of penicillin. In fact, in WW2, wounded Australian soldiers were given tea tree oil to prevent infections.

My friend, who has the most sensitive skin, got athlete's foot on her last vacation. She said she had spent her days in the hotel's swimming pool – a breeding ground for the fungus. She called me the minute she noticed it, to ask what she should put on her fungal infection. I told her to use tea tree oil, which she found in a local health store. Three days after that, she sent me a picture of her freshly pedicured feet without any sign of the ugly infection.

Native to: Australia

Description: The pointed leaves of the tea tree, and especially their essential oil, are the most effective antiseptic found in nature. First officially confirmed as effective in Australia in 1923, tea tree is a traditional Aboriginal remedy that has been intensively researched since the sixties. The leaves can be crushed and inhaled for coughs, or used as infusions for skin problems. Tea tree has been an effective healer of many infections: skin, oral, gynecological, and even chronic.

Main Components: Volatile oil

Medicinal Actions:
Antiseptic
Antifungal
Antibacterial
Antiviral
Immune Stimulant

Main Uses:
Treats Cystitis
Treats Skin Infections (ringworm, athlete's foot)
Relieves Boils and Acne
Treats Vaginal Infections
Treats Gum Disease
Sore Throat Gargle
Relieves Coughs
Helps Treat Chronic Fatigue Syndrome

Parts Used: The leaves

Practical use: Good for making essential oils, infusions, and creams.

Safety Precautions: Do not consume tea tree internally. Also, don't apply tea tree oil topically if it is undiluted, as it can cause irritation.

THYME
(Thymus vulgaris)

Thymol is a powerful volatile oil found in thyme. This chemical compound plays an important part in hand sanitizers, mouthwashes, and acne meditation today. In the 19th century, Victorian nurses used to soak their bandages in thyme-diluted water to stop infections from spreading. Before the modern era of refrigerators, monasteries depended on thyme to store their food without it spoiling.

A few winters back, the weather was deceptively warm. I

was out Christmas shopping a few days in advance, so I thought leaving my coat in the car would be a good idea. When sweaty skin and low temperatures mix, chest infection is almost guaranteed. My thyme syrup helped me power through the coughs and the infection. By the time Christmas rolled around, I was sipping on champagne.

Native to: Southern Europe

Description: Thyme is more than just the herb you use to spice up your pork chops or roast chicken. It is the superstar of your windowsill garden, not only because of its uncanny ability to make holiday food delicious – though that is undeniable – but also because of its powerful medicinal properties. For centuries, it has been used as a cough remedy; and when used to make syrup, it can battle serious respiratory issues. It is also great for infections and as an immune-boosting tonic.

Main Components: Volatile oil

Medicinal Actions:
Antiseptic
Expectorant
Tonic
Antioxidant
Antispasmodic

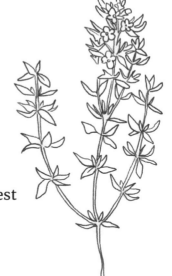

Main Uses:
Treats Asthma Symptoms
Relieves Coughs and Respiratory Issues
Effective in Dealing with Chest Infections
Tonic for the Immune System
Helps Expel Worms
Relieves Bites and Stings

Parts Used: The aerial parts (that grow above ground)

Practical use: Another great herb for making an essential oil, syrup, infusion, or tincture.

Safety Precautions: Thyme can slow down blood clotting

and may increase bleeding, so be wary of how you use this herb if undergoing a surgery. Taking thyme with anticoagulant medications is not recommended.

VALERIAN
(Valeriana officinalis)

Derived from the Latin "valere" which translates as "to be well," valerian is one of the most powerful herbs around. This is an herb that knocks down stress, aids sleep, and soothes the being. In war-torn Sarajevo (Bosnia and Herzegovina), back in 1993, doctors depended on Valeriana officinalis to treat traumatized soldiers. This was at a time when medical supplies were unavailable. Valerian has been a popular relaxant since Roman times, and studies have found it to be as effective as sedative drugs such as oxazepam.

Our friends have a beautiful five-year-old boy. When he was three and a half years old, they moved to a new apartment, and he started experiencing trouble falling asleep. He would wake up after ten minutes and cry for an hour. His pediatrician had prescribed a medication, but it wasn't helpful. I suggested an herbal valerian supplement. Three days after that, they called to thank me for restoring their beauty sleep again.

Native to: Europe, Northern Asia

Description: Thanks to its non-addictive and relaxing properties, valerian has become one of the safest and most effective sedatives in the world. Its rhizome and root are also used for treating epilepsy because they decrease mental over-activity. It is recommended to those people who cannot "switch off" because it has a powerful calming effect. It is the perfect addition to your first-aid kit for when you need a booster to bring back the feel-good vibes. When combined with other herbs, valerian can also help lower blood pressure.

Main Components: Volatile oil, alkaloids, iridoids

Medicinal Actions:
Relaxant
Sedative
Antispasmodic

Anxiety Relief

Main Uses:
Improves Sleep
Relieves Stress
Relieves Anxiety
Relieves Panic and Tremor
Reduces Sweating
Relaxes Contracting Muscles
Helps with Neck and Shoulder Tension

Parts Used: The root and rhizome

Practical use: Prepare this amazing herb as a tincture, tablets, decoction, or a powder to extract the benefits.

Safety Precautions: Generally safe for both internal and external use. However, valerian slows down the central nervous system, so it can be harmful if taken with anesthetics or before and after surgery. It can also do the reverse, and act as a stimulant in a small percentage of the population, particularly the clinically hyperactive.

WITCH HAZEL
(Hamamelis virginiana)

Originally called "The Golden Treasure," witch hazel was the first mass-marketed herbal remedy in America. It was developed in 1846 by an American pharmacist (T. T. Pond), and marketed as Pond's Extract (Gartrell, 2000). Despite its name, witch hazel has nothing to do with the occult or with stirring up potions. It originates from the Middle English "wicke" which means "lively" or "bendable." Wicke is a word used to describe the Y-shaped stick used in the ancient technique of searching for underground water. But even if it does not refer to witches, that doesn't mean it lacks magical prowess. When it comes to soothing irritated skin, cleaning wounds, and reducing inflammation, this plant has been found, in studies, to be an effective treatment (Wolff & Kieser, 2007).

A small bottle with distilled witch hazel water is always in my first-aid kit. When we were visiting France's countryside, I fell off my bike and hurt my knee quite badly. I told you I was clumsy! The injury was so bad that I needed stitches. I cleaned my knee with my witch hazel water that was in the kit in my backpack. When I finally got to the hospital, three hours later, the nurse told me that she had never seen anyone do such a good job at cleaning a wound before. I told her it was nothing but some witch hazel, and she was quite impressed with my herbal knowledge.

Native to: Canada, Eastern USA

Description: Yellow flowers that bloom in the freezing winter? This may have been the first hint to the Native North Americans that there was something mysterious about this plant. Whatever force persuaded them to try the mystical plant, we surely must thank it. The Food and Drug Administration approves witch hazel as a natural non-prescription drug. A powerful remedy for inflammations, wound cleaning, skin issues, and insect stings, this plant is versatile enough to bring benefits to several elements of your life.

Main Components: Tannins, volatile oil (the leaves only), flavonoids, bitters

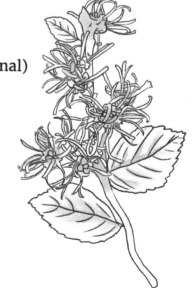

Medicinal Actions:
Anti-inflammatory
Astringent
Stops Bleeding (internal and external)

Main Uses:
Protects and Heals Broken Skin
Cleans Wounds
Treats Eczema
Repairs Damaged Facial Veins
Tightens Distended Veins
Eyewash for Eye Inflammation
Treats Diarrhea
Reduces Heavy Menstrual Flow
Soothes Insect Bites

Parts Used: The leaves and bark

Practical use: This is an old favorite of mine and you can prepare it as a tincture, distilled witch hazel, infusion, and as an ointment.

Safety Precautions: Though generally safe for everyone, a special precaution should be taken with dosages, as large amounts of witch hazel, consumed internally, may cause liver issues.

These 12 herbs cover a wide range of medicinal uses and form the ultimate natural first-aid kit. Unless you absolutely need to choose a conventional aggressive medication (sometimes garlic will not do the trick, and you will need a pharmaceutical antibiotic), I suggest you pack the herbal remedies into your handy medicine bag and keep this bag with you at all times.

Other Essential Herbs for the Home Apothecary

Apart from the plants that can practice first aid, many other herbs are also full of medicinal properties for your overall health. From agrimony to yarrow, here are the essential herbs that you should understand and master if you want to practice your herbal healing skills. For centuries, all these herbs and plants have been pressed, steeped, or infused to aid in the healing of the human body.

AGRIMONY
(Agrimonia eupatoria)

We have come a long way since placing agrimony sprigs under the bed for a good night's sleep, as British folklore dictates. We've also improved since the Anglo-Saxonian way of boiling agrimony in milk for erectile purposes. As Michael Drayton, an English poet who lived from 1563–1631, said, "agrimony is really an 'all-heal'." Many studies later, we think the same way! From staunching bleeding to being used as a tonic to aid digestion, this versatile plant can support our health in many different ways.

Whenever my daughter has diarrhea, I prepare agrimony tea and give it to her twice a day. The next day, the symptoms are almost gone, and her digestion is much improved

Native to: Europe

Description: Herbalists dry the aerial parts and the seeds of this mildly aromatic plant. Agrimony has a long history as a wound healer, thanks to its clot-forming properties, but it is also widely used as a tonic for treating diarrhea and supporting digestion. In Traditional Chinese Medicine, agrimony is the go-to herb for stopping bleeding and heavy menstruation.
When combined with other herbs, it can also treat urinary tract and kidney conditions.

Main Components: Flavonoids, coumarins, polysaccharides, bitters, tannins, vitamins B and K

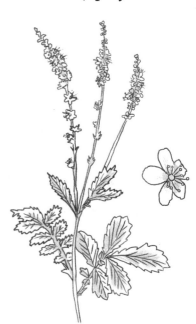

Medicinal Actions:
Anti-inflammatory
Diuretic
Astringent
Tonic
Cholagogue
Hemostatic

Main Uses:
Heals Wounds
Coagulates Blood
Relieves Diarrhea
Increases Blood Flood
Supports Digestion
Liver Tonic
Helpful for Rashes and Acne

Parts Used: The parts that grow above the ground (stems, leaves, flowers)

Practical use: The tea is probably the fastest and easiest to make but you can also prepare a tincture, compresses, and eye baths to treat discharge and inflammation.

Safety Precautions: Avoid agrimony during pregnancy and breastfeeding. Do not consume more than 3 g a day, internally. Agrimony lowers blood sugar levels, so avoid taking agrimony with medications for diabetes.

ALOE VERA
(Aloe barbadensis)

Aloe vera is one of the oldest medicinal herbs on this planet. As legends report, the ancient Greek philosopher, Aristotle, advised Alexander the Great, a powerful ruler of Macedonia, to conquer an African island to stock up on aloe vera supplies. This would allegedly cure his wounded soldiers. More than 2200 years later, Japanese soldiers in WW2 also used this plant's gel to heal their wounds in a natural way. Aloe vera may be an old-time plant, but it surely gives us a timeless cure!

Last Christmas, I was so busy in the kitchen preparing supper I burned my hand quite badly on the stove. When my husband saw the burn, he was concerned for me and thought that it would leave a huge scar. I treated my hand with aloe vera gel for a few days, and voila! The mark faded rapidly and disappeared into the mist, never to be seen again.

Native to: North Africa, Southern Europe

Description: Aloe vera is extensively cultivated as a potted plant worldwide, and it is one of the most commonly used plants for beauty and skin treatments. Cleopatra, the ruler of Egypt from 52–31 BC, the real-life Aphrodite, attributed her timeless beauty to aloe. So, it is clear that aloe was being used a very long time ago. Aloe vera has two main medicinal uses: a gel from the leaves that is used for healing wounds and treating burns; and the dried, powdered, yellow sap from the leaves, used as a bitter laxative for constipation. Herbalists cut the leaves open to scrape the gel, and then they drain them to collect the bitter liquid.

Main Components: Anthraquinones, tannins, resins, Aloectin B, polysaccharides

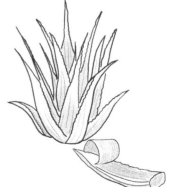

Medicinal Actions:
Heals
Laxative
Emollient
Stimulates Bile Secretion

Main Uses:

Heals Wounds
Treats Burn
Relieves Sunburn
Treats Ulcers
Relieves Irritable Bowel Syndrome (IBS)
Alleviates Various Skin Conditions

Parts Used: The leaves, broken for the gel and drained for the liquid

Practical use: Make the famous aloe gel, juice, or tincture to extract the medicines you desire.

Safety Precautions: People who are allergic to garlic and onion may also be allergic to aloe vera. Do not apply to severe burns and deep cuts, as it may have an adverse effect.

ANGELICA
(Angelica officinalis)

With over 4000 years of use in Traditional Chinese Medicine, Angelica is one of the oldest medicinal herbs popular among natural-healing practitioners worldwide. The name is derived from a 17th-century monk's dream in which St. Michael told him to use this plant to cure the bubonic plague. It was considered an "angel" on earth and chronicles report that people at that time believed that chewing angelica root all day would make them immune to the plague.

One of my closest friends began struggling with her menstrual cycle after giving birth. She tried all sorts of hormonal medications prescribed by her gynecologist, but nothing did the trick. I recommended she give an angelica infusion a shot. After a couple of weeks, everything went back to functioning normally.

Native to: The Northern Hemisphere (subarctic and temperate regions)

Description: The genus Angelica contains about 60 different species with Norwegian, American, and Chinese angelica being the most popular ones. Angelica is a tall plant with bipinnate leaves and green or whiteish flowers grouped together into large umbels. Used for medicinal properties, angelica is a powerful natural tonic that treats many conditions specific to women, as well as heartburn, anemia, intestinal gas, and circulation. It is also used to treat hair loss because it causes increased circulation in the scalp. In China, dong quai angelica (*Angelica sinensis*) is mainly used for its property of causing uterine contractions and as a natural gynecological supplement.

Main Components: Volatile oils, ferulic acid, coumarins, polyacetylenes, phytosterols

Medicinal Actions:
Antispasmodic
Anti-inflammatory
Blood Thinner

Tonic
Stomachic

Main Uses:
Helps Uterine Contraction
Supports Healthy Menstrual Flow
Used for Treating Anemia, or Other
Blood-loss Conditions
Improves Circulation of the Abdomen,
Feet, and Hands
Aids Conception
Reduces Hair Loss

Parts Used: The root, fruit, rhizome, and seeds

Practical use: Tincture, infusion, tonic wine

Safety Precautions: Do not take angelica internally during pregnancy, as it can cause uterine contractions.

BASIL
(Ocimum basilicum)

Although most people usually make use of basil for culinary, not medicinal purposes, this plant is quite the healer. A powerful traditional remedy for inflammation, colds, and even snakebites, basil has many different health uses. For those who care deeply for their skin, studies have found basil to be loaded with anti-aging properties that prevent skin from drooping or sagging.

When my aforementioned friend was pregnant, she suffered from severe nausea. Even today, years later, she still thanks me for recommending basil juice to her. It made her mornings bearable, and after using basil for a time, she was able to enjoy food again.

Native to: India

Description: Basil is an herb you'll find used in kitchens all over the world, but it has also been shown to have a tremendous effect on our overall health. Extensively grown in Central and South America, and as a potted plant throughout the world, basil is an aromatic, annual herb of the mint family. Depending on the species (holy, sweet), the taste of the leaves varies, but they are all used for similar medicinal purposes. The key benefit of this plant is that it lowers blood glucose levels, so it is a common supplement for regulating diabetes. Sweet basil, in particular, has powerful therapeutic properties and is quite successful in easing nausea.

Main Components: Flavonoids, volatile oil, triterpene, saponins, polyphenols

Medicinal Actions:
Analgesic
Adaptogenic
Anti-inflammatory
Therapeutic
Antispasmodic
Anti-aging

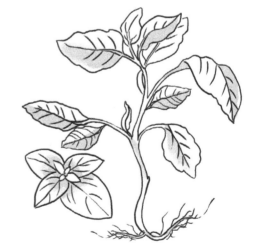

Main Uses:
Lowers Blood Sugar
Reduces Fever
Relieves Nausea
Treats Stomach Cramps
Supports Digestion
Tonic to Improve Vitality
Relieves the Skin from Insect Bites

Parts Used: The aerial parts (that grow above ground)

Practical use: You probably already use this in your culinary recipes but you can also make a basil tonic, juice, powder rub or a decoction.

Safety Precautions: Basil extracts and oils can slow down blood clotting. Avoid consumption if suffering from a bleeding disorder, as well as before and after surgeries.

BLACK COHOSH
(Cimicifuga racemosa)

The popular Eclectic physician of the 19th century, John King, used to teach his students about black cohosh, his favorite remedy. Primarily known as "macrotys," black cohosh was the key remedy in Eclectic practices for treating chronic rheumatoid conditions.

Although I haven't had the chance to explore fully the benefits of this herb myself, my mother swears to its efficiency. She has been suffering from kidney issues her whole life, and she claims that black cohosh tincture is what keeps her out of the hospital.

Native to: Eastern USA, Canada

Description: Black cohosh is a powerful Native American supplement that has been used for women's conditions, such as menopause and painful menstrual cycles, for a long time. The root of the plant is the only part that is used and, although the taste is acrid and bitter, this natural remedy is still popular for treating kidney and rheumatic issues. You can find black cohosh growing widely and wildly in Europe, thanks to its seed propagation. You can also find this plant under the name of "black snake root" or "rattle top."

Main Components: Isoflavones, triterpenes, isoferulic acid

Medicinal Actions:
Sedative
Anti-inflammatory
Estrogenic
Antirheumatic
Expectorant

Main Uses:
Used for Treating Menopausal Symptoms
Relieves Painful Periods
Treats Rheumatoid Arthritis and Other Similar Issues
Treats Tinnitus (Ringing in the Ears)
Supports Kidney Health

Parts Used: The root

Practical use: Try making tinctures, decoctions, or tablets according to the chapter "Harnessing the Essence of Herbs."

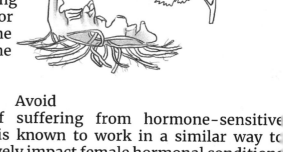

Safety Precautions: Avoid during pregnancy and if suffering from hormone-sensitive conditions. Black cohosh is known to work in a similar way to estrogen, and it can negatively impact female hormonal conditions such as endometriosis, uterine and ovarian cancer, fibroids, etc.

CATNIP
(Nepeta cataria)

If you own a cat, then you probably are aware of this herb and the effect it has on your feline buddy – it makes cats roll, flip, growl, meow and, in the end – zone out. With a slightly different but also sedating intensity, this herb also affects humans. An old hangman's tale tells of how calming and relaxing the effect of catnip is. To endure his profession, the hangman used to drink a catnap (pun intended) tea before work, so he would not struggle as much with the ethical dilemma of his profession.

When my daughter was little, I used to give her catnip tea to restore balance to her colicky and upset tummy. This was especially beneficial if consumed around bedtime, as it used to promote a good night's sleep. For both of us!

Native to: Europe

Description: Born in Europe but naturalized in North America, catnip is an aromatic herb that commonly grows in higher-altitude and wayside areas. It has heart-shaped leaves and white flowers with purple dots. The flowering parts are used for medicinal purposes, mostly for settling an upset stomach or providing relief from colic. Thanks to its mild and non-bitter taste, catnip is good for treating infant, child and adult colic, anxiety, stress headache, and stomach trouble. It is also excellent in fighting colds and fevers because it encourages sweating. Sweetened with some honey, it can make a safe sedating remedy for children.

Main Components: Tannins, iridoids, volatile oil

Medicinal Actions:
Soothes Nerves
Encourages Sweating
Sedative
Relaxant
Anti-inflammatory
Spasmolytic
Antidiarrheal
Carminative

Main Uses:
Relief from Indigestion
Relief from Colic and Cramping
Reduces Fever, Cold, Flu
Treats Headaches
Lowers Anxiety
Reduces Rheumatism-related Pain when Applied as a Rub

Parts Used: The aerial parts (that grow above ground)

Practical use: Works perfectly as a tea, tincture, tonic, rub and compress.

Safety Precautions: Considered possibly unsafe for children, when taken in large doses. Should not be taken during pregnancy or breastfeeding. Avoid if planning on taking anesthetics or if suffering from pelvic inflammatory disease.

CHAMOMILE
(Chamomilla recutita)

Both Roman and German chamomiles are popular herbs used for their therapeutic properties. But there is a lot more than meets the eye with these well-known flowers. They do much more than simply soothe the nerves. I have found out that the herb penetrates deeply below the skin's surface, when applied topically, which makes chamomile an excellent anti-inflammatory agent.

If I don't savor a hot cuppa of chamomile tea before going to bed, I feel I cannot fall asleep. It relaxes and soothes me deeply, which is especially appreciated on those hectic days when all I want to do is unwind.

Native to: Europe

Description: German chamomile is one of the most widely used natural remedies. It is easy to cultivate as it is not demanding and thrives in temperate conditions. Chamomile has been the go-to natural supplement for herbalists in many eras, thanks to its soothing and relieving properties. The sweet, aromatic, white flowers with yellow centers offer an apple-like taste, perfect for tea. Roman chamomile is a closely related herb that offers similar medicinal benefits.

Main Components: Volatile oil, coumarins, flavonoids, bitter glycosides

Medicinal Actions:
Relaxant
Anti-inflammatory

Carminative
Antispasmodic
Antiallergenic

Main Uses:
Treats Indigestion
Relieves an Upset Stomach (bloating, acidity, gas)
Promotes Sleep

Eases Muscle Cramps
Eases Menstrual Cramping
Relieves Hay Fever and Asthma
Externally Useful for Itchy or Sore Skin

Parts Used: The flower heads (fresh or dried)

Practical use: A warm tea is very suitable. Even tinctures, essential oils and creams are great choices.

Safety Precautions: German chamomile is generally safe for everyone, but there are some precautions. Birth control pills, estrogen, and sedatives all interact with chamomile, so avoid using them together, or consult with your physician.

CHICKWEED
(Stellaria media)

Chickweed is one of the most popular folk medicines. Well-known herbalists used to recommend it for treating skin conditions, pulmonary diseases, and as a remedy for mange (a parasitic skin disease). For the Ainu, the indigenous people of Japan, it was a go-to herb for bruises and bone aches. Although there isn't much scientific evidence to back this up, herbal enthusiasts swear by its incredible effects. Chickweed is bursting with iron, so it makes a great supplement for those suffering from anemia.

When my daughter was three years old, she was overcome by a severe case of eczema. She had struggled with itchy skin before that as well, but this was especially irritating. I didn't buy any conventional creams to relieve her itchiness. Instead, I used my homemade chickweed remedy and applied it daily. Not only did we manage to relieve her itchiness, but we also reversed the condition within a week.

Native to: Europe, Asia

Description: Small perennial with white flowers, oval leaves, and hairy stems. Although generally perceived as troublesome, chickweed is often found growing in wastelands and is quite a beneficial herb. Loaded with anti-inflammatory properties, this natural supplement is mainly used for treating irritated skin and, in some cases, extreme itchiness. Be mindful that, if consumed in larger quantities, chickweed can induce vomiting and cause diarrhea.

Main Components: Flavonoids, triterpenoid saponins, vitamin C, carboxylic acids

Medicinal Actions:
Anti-inflammatory
Emollient
Soothing Ointment
Anti-obesity Actions

Main Uses:
Treats Irritated Skin
Reduces Itchiness
Relieves Eczema, Nettle Rash, Venous Ulcers
Used for Baby's Diaper Rash
Relieves Stomach and Bowel Issues
Reduces Rheumatic Inflammation
Helps Maintain Weight

Parts Used: The aerial parts (the parts growing above ground)

Practical use: Makes a great cream, bath infusion and tea.

Safety Precautions: Generally safe to consume, but in medicinal amounts only. In high doses, chickweed causes vomiting and nausea. Avoid during pregnancy.

DANDELION
(Taraxacum officinale)

Did you know that the milky white part of the dandelion stalk produces natural latex? During WW2, when the world was facing shortages in rubber supplies due to all the military needs, the world was forced to start looking for a natural alternative. And they found that alternative in dandelions. Or in their white sap, to be precise. But while your body may not have much use for dandelion latex, know that the same milky juice is quite effective for treating skin infections such as ringworm or eczema.

I absolutely love dandelion! In addition to making tablets and tinctures, I love incorporating the leaves into salads for lunch. I often struggle with high blood pressure, so this is another thing that helps me keep it in check.

Native to: Europe, Asia

Description: Dandelion is more than just a fun flower for kids to blow floaties. It is loaded with beneficial properties that support our health. Growing almost everywhere in the world and normally considered by the population to be a weed, dandelion is one of the easiest medicinal herbs to come by. Whether you choose to use the young leaves for a diuretic salad or harvest them later for tea, juices, or tinctures, this plant with yellow flowers, hollow stalks and basal leaves will cleanse your body from the inside out.

Main Components: Triterpenes, sesquiterpene lactones, polysaccharides, potassium – leaf and root. There are carotenoids and coumarins in the leaves, and phenolic acids, calcium, and taraxacoside hidden within the roots.

Medicinal Actions:
Bitter
Diuretic
Detoxifier
Anti-inflammatory

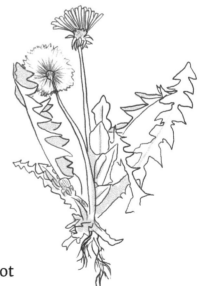

Main Uses:
Treats High Blood Pressure – leaf
Reduces Bodily Fluids – leaf
Stimulates the Liver – leaf
Treats Constipation – root
Reduces Local Inflammation – root
Treats Eczema – root
Good for Arthritic Issues – root
Stimulates Insulin Production – root

Parts Used: The root and leaves

Practical use: You can go almost any route you wish with the easily found and very beneficial dandelion! My suggestions are tonics, juices, teas, tinctures, tablets, and consumed raw in salad (leaf only).

Safety Precautions: Generally safe, but in medicinal dose only. People with eczema are at higher risk of being allergic to dandelion, so do your due diligence before consuming. Also dandelion is known to interact with antibiotics and can change the way that certain antibiotics react in the body.

ELDER
(Sambucus nigra; Sambucus canadensis)

If you search the mists of 19th- and 20th-century folklore, you will definitely encounter elder. People believed that the Elder Mother, the elder guardian in Scandinavian and English folklore, inhabited the elder tree, so they always approached it with respect when gathering their medicines.

Today, elderflowers and elderberries still support our health in many mystical and magical ways. A couple of elderflower tea cuppas a day is my go-to remedy for slaying annoying seasonal allergies. Start consuming it a few months before the season hits and you might lower your sensitivity and the severity of your allergies.

Native to: Europe

Description: You can find elder trees in most parts of Europe, thriving in the woods and in open areas. Its flowers and berries are loaded with medicinal properties that can relieve us from respiratory issues, purge cold and flu, and even support the removal of waste products by encouraging sweating and increasing urine production. If you dry the berries and make a decoction, you've got yourself a mild natural laxative. There are two black-berried varieties used medicinally: *S. nigra*, native to Europe and *S. canadensis*, native to North America. Both have the same uses.

Main Components: Flavonoids, tannins, anthocyanins, volatile oil, triterpenes, mucilage

Medicinal Actions:
Anti-inflammatory
Antiviral

Diuretic
Cleanses Mucus

Main Uses:
Treats Respiratory Infections
Lowers Cold and Flu Symptoms
Reduces Allergy Symptoms
Encourages Sweating
Controls Diabetes
Lowers Blood Pressure

Parts Used: The flowering tops and berries

Practical use: Make a tincture, tea, infusion or cream, depending on your needs and your mood.

Safety Precautions: Elderberries are considered not suitable for children younger than 12 years old. Elderflowers can cause vomiting and nausea if taken in high doses, and they can also interact with diabetes medications.

FENNEL
(Foeniculum vulgare)

Fennel is one of the three main herbs used in the traditional, often banned, Absinthe recipe. It is also one of the nine herbs that were sacred to the Anglo-Saxons, the Germanic peoples who inhabited England in the 5th century. During medieval times, fennel was used to keep bad spirits away; this may or may not have been successful but, regardless, fennel still boasts powerful insect-repellent qualities.

Speaking of repellants, fennel is the perfect remedy for purging bad bacteria from the gut and one of the most effective natural digestive aids. My husband, who often struggles with digestive issues, benefits especially from fennel tea. He drinks a cup every couple of days as a preventive measure. I also used a fennel infusion as an eyewash when I was going through an annoyingly itchy allergy.
Native to: Mediterranean

Description: Cultivated in all temperate regions throughout the world, fennel is an aromatic plant with feather-like leaves, yellow flowers, and oval seeds. You've probably used these ingredients in cooking. When it comes to digestion, these little oval goodies, packed with volatile oil, work like magic. Apart from treating stomach-related issues, fennel seeds are also beneficial when used as an eyewash or for relief from conjunctivitis.

Main Components: Volatile oil, coumarins, sterols, flavonoids

Medicinal Actions:
Digestive Aid
Carminative
Antispasmodic

Main Uses:
Treats Bloating
Stimulates Appetite
Increases Breast Milk Production
Relieves Stomach-Related Issues in Infants, in Low Doses
Relieves Conjunctivitis
Relieves Menopausal Symptoms
Supports Weight Loss

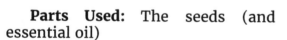

Parts Used: The seeds (and essential oil)

Practical use: Treat yourself with teas, capsules, tinctures, infusions and try fennel in culinary dishes.

Safety Precautions: Avoid with estrogen and birth control pills.

GINGER
(Zingiber officinale)

Ginger has been one of the most popular herbs for medicinal and culinary purposes; there has been a consistent demand for the plant throughout the centuries. The first record dates back to Confucius, who was known to eat this fragrant Indian staple with every meal. If you suffer from indigestion, you may want to consider doing the same, as studies find ginger to be quite effective in the stomach-emptying process (Bodagh et al., 2019).

A gingery infusion is my go-to morning drink. I have been drinking this for years to boost my immune system and support my weight maintenance goal.

Native to: Asia

Description: Ginger is more than just an aromatic staple in Asian cuisine. Rich in a volatile oil and packed with a pungent lemony taste, the rhizome of this plant is a must-have supplement for anyone looking for a natural approach to treating health issues. Thanks to its warming and stimulating properties, ginger has many medicinal uses. Supporting digestive health and relieving migraines and headaches are among the most common ones.

Main Components: Volatile oil, oleoresin

Medicinal Actions:
Anti-inflammatory
Digestive Stimulant
Circulatory Stimulant
Antiviral
Anti-emetic

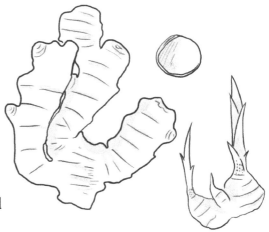

Main Uses:
Supports Iron Absorption, Good for Anemia
Treats Indigestion and Supports Gastric Emptying
Reduces Muscle Pain
Relieves Morning Sickness and Motion Sickness
Relieves Symptoms of Spondylosis
Improves Circulation in Feet, Hands
Remedy for Chilblains
Remedy for Flu, Cough, and Respiratory Problems
Controls Fevers
Relieves Headaches

Parts Used: The rhizome

Practical use: One of my favorites, on a cold winter night, when made into a heartwarming tea. But also useful as infusions, tinctures, capsules, and essential oils.

Safety Precautions: Ginger is safe for both internal and external use. However, since it increases the risk of bleeding, this plant interacts with medications that reduce blood clotting and should not be taken along with such drugs.

GINKGO
(Ginkgo biloba)

The ginkgo, the only living species in a genus of ancient, extinct trees, is in high demand as an herbal supplement. In early times, it was the magic bullet for improving memory and other age-related issues. Scientific evidence suggests that ginkgo may slow down the progression of Alzheimer's disease (Salleh, 2014), although that is not all this wonderful plant can accomplish. Ginkgo is most beneficial if used for glaucoma or blood circulation issues.

When my cousin's son was diagnosed with asthma, I suggested they give him a ginkgo remedy when the symptoms intensified. They say that he started feeling better after the first couple of sips. I haven't tried this myself, but many people claim that ginkgo has an incredible effect on asthmatic patients.

Native to: China

Description: It is believed that the ginkgo species is more than 190 million years old and that it is actually the oldest type of tree on earth. Although the therapeutic leaves have been an age-old medicine in native China, their beneficial properties have been made known to the world more recently. Research into this beautiful tree is just beginning. Ginkgo is one of the few herbs that crosses the blood-brain barrier (Liang et al., 2020) and this is the reason it is able to improve memory and circulation in the brain. It is also used as a relief from wheezing.

Main Components: Flavonoids, bilobalides, ginkgolides

Medicinal Actions:
Anti-inflammatory
Tonic for Circulation
Anti-allergenic
Antispasmodic
Anti-asthmatic

Main Uses:
Reduces Phlegm
Relieves Wheezing
Improves Blood Circulation,
Especially to the Brain
Relieves Asthmatic Symptoms

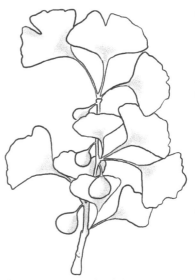

Parts Used: The leaves and seeds

Practical use: Try tonics, tinctures, decoctions, fluid extracts and tablets to see what suits your body best.

Safety Precautions: Ginkgo leaves are safe to consume in appropriate doses, but the seeds are not recommended for internal consumption. Consuming more than ten seeds can cause a weak pulse, serious difficulty in breathing, shock, and seizures. Not safe during pregnancy and not recommended if taking Ibuprofen, as it can slow down blood clotting.

GINSENG
(Panax ginseng)

If you visit the Geumsan region in South Korea, you may hear a 1500-year-old tale about a boy named Kang. When praying for his ill mother on Mount Jinak, a guardian spirit told Kang to look for a plant with three red fruits, take it home, and feed his mother the root. Soon after feeding his mother the root, the magical tea got his mother out of bed. The plant, as you may have guessed, was ginseng. Kang devoted his life to cultivating this magical plant and, in doing so, paved the region's path to becoming Korea's largest source of ginseng.

A dear friend of mine had liver cell damage (non-alcoholic fatty liver disease) and managed to reverse the condition within a couple of weeks by drinking ginseng tea every day. I wonder whether

Kang's mother suffered from the same illness. Regardless, studies support that this herb has a great effect on the liver.

Native to: North and South Korea, Northeastern China, Eastern Russia

Description: As one of the most popular Chinese perennial plants, ginseng has been used as an herbal medicine for thousands of years. Difficult to cultivate and rarely found in the wild, this plant's root not easy to get your hands on. However, if you can manage to find it, ginseng can bring you tons of benefits. Excellent at improving stamina, ginseng is a popular supplement among athletes. It also serves as a male aphrodisiac. Although it is mainly used in Western societies for reducing stress, ginseng is also a powerful weapon for boosting the immune system and liver function.

Main Components: Panaxans, triterpenoid saponins, sesquiterpenes, acetylenic compounds

Medicinal Actions:
Tonic
Adaptogen
Stimulant
Hormonal Balancer

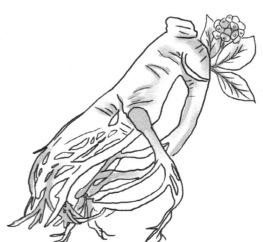

Main Uses:
Lowers Stress
Improves Stamina
Improves the Immune Function
Supports Liver Health
Reduces Nervousness and Anxiety

Parts Used: The root

Practical use: Ginseng works well in tonics, soups, and capsules.

Safety Precautions: Avoid taking in combination with diabetes medications as it can affect blood sugar levels. Since ginseng can also raise blood pressure, avoid taking it in combination with caffeine. It also interacts with depression medications and Warfarin.

GOLDENSEAL
(Hydrastis canadensis)

You may have heard the urban legend that consuming goldenseal before giving a urine sample can cover up the presence of recreational drugs. This probably stems from the 1900s novel Stringtown on the Pike, in which goldenseal causes false positives for strychnine poisoning. While I cannot comment on whether the writer, John Uri Lloyd, an herbal pharmacist himself, knew that this was only a myth, scientists had already dismissed the urban legend. Goldenseal can help you detox from cannabis, but it may not help you pass a drug test. Goldenseal will actually support metabolic flushing, which will lead to more THC in the urine.

When late fall rolls over, my annual sinus complications arise. When I was younger, I used to struggle with infusions and inhalations until I discovered that goldenseal extract was actually the most beneficial cure. I start consuming goldenseal in late summer and, as summer rolls along, I do not notice a single intense symptom.

Native to: North America

Description: This old Cherokeean remedy, goldenseal, was known as the cure-all herb for the Native Americans in the 19th century. The traditional use of this plant involved combining it with bear fat and applying it to repel insects, but it was also perfect for treating ulcers, wounds, and sores. Today, goldenseal is a rare and even endangered species that has many different practical uses. Goldenseal is perfect for stimulating the uterine muscles, thanks to the high alkaloid content, but is equally effective in lowering fat levels and maintaining a glucose balance in the blood.

Main Components: Isoquinoline alkaloids, resin, volatile oil

Medicinal Actions:
Tonic
Antibacterial
Uterine Stimulant
Anti-inflammatory

Main Uses:
Stops Internal Bleeding
Reduces Heavy Menstrual or Postpartum Bleeding
Stabilizes Blood Glucose
Remedy for the Mucous Membrane (Eyes, Nose, Throat, Ears, Stomach)

Parts Used: The rhizome

Practical use: This one is perfectly fine as a tincture, infusion, powder, decoction and capsules. Capsules can keep for a long time, without becoming spoiled.

Safety Precautions: Not recommended for children or during pregnancy and breastfeeding.

HAWTHORN
(Crataegus spp.)

Humankind has a long-standing bond with this plant. It extends from meeting fairy queens by hawthorn bushes, to the legend of Jesus' uncle planting the Holy Thorn of Glastonbury in Britain, and to the British Queen who decorates her Christmas table each year with a Holy Hawthorn sprig. It is known to soften the heart and be perfect for healing from grief. But that is not why it is known as "food for the heart." Studies suggest that hawthorn is the ideal natural supplement for reducing oxidative stress and is the best aid for supporting the cardiovascular system (Wu et al., 2020).

I frequently consume hawthorn tonic for lowering blood pressure. I'm not a big fan of its bitter taste, but I can swear by its effect on normalizing the old ticker.

Native to: Great Britain

Description: This tree sports red berries and grows along roadsides. Oftentimes, the plant is mistakenly considered poisonous. Although it doesn't taste great in a berry parfait, it will surely energize the cells of your heart. Primarily, it is used for treating angina or heart irregularities, thanks to its power to dilate and relax the arteries. It is equally effective for improving memory and the blood flow to the brain, especially when taken in combination with ginkgo.

Main   Components: Coumarins,   polyphenols, b i o f l a v o n o i d s , triterpenoids,   amines, proanthocyanins

Medicinal Actions:
Antioxidant
Circulatory Tonic
Cardiotonic

Main Uses:
Lowers Blood Pressure
Reduces Angina Symptoms
Increases Blood Flow to the Muscles
Increases Blood Flow to the Brain
Treats Coronary Artery Diseases
Great for Normalizing Heartbeat

Parts Used: The flowering tops and berries

Practical use: Aim for a decoction, tonic, tincture, infusion or make tablets.

Safety Precautions: Not recommended for those who take heart medications. It can also interact with drugs for high blood pressure, so consult with a physician before using it. Avoid during pregnancy and breastfeeding.

HOPS
(Humulus lupulus)

First used for brewing beer in the 16th century in England, this herb was considered by the parliament of that time as "the wicked herb." Since becoming an integral ingredient in one of the most consumed beverages on Earth, scientists have started exploring the effects this herb has on our health over time (Kyrou et al., 2017). And the results don't lie! Hops can be quite beneficial. Consume hops regularly, and you will not have problems falling asleep, or with anxiety.

I drink hops infusions when I need to unwind mentally. I don't usually suffer from insomnia but, when I do, I can be up and turning all night, unable to fall asleep. When this severe condition pays me a visit, I brew myself some hops tea, add a dash of valerian to it, and sleep like a baby.

Native to: Europe, Asia

Description: You may not have seen climbing hop plants often, but you have surely tasted this herb many times before. Hops give beer its bitter and characteristic taste. The hop plant is a member of the *cannabis* family, and hops have similar sedative and sleep-inducing properties. They can also help relax your muscles and even bring an estrogenic effect.

Main Components: Volatile oil, bitters, flavonoids, estrogenic substances, polyphenolic tannins

Medicinal Actions:
Sedative
Antispasmodic
Contains   Aromatic   Bitter
Compounds
Soporific

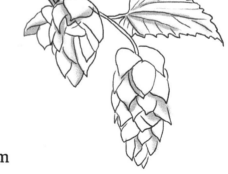

Main Uses:
Treats Insomnia
Lowers Excitability
Relaxes Muscles
Stimulates the Digestive System
Reduces Tension and Stress

Parts Used: The strobiles (the conelike female flowers)

Practical use: Use in an infusion, tincture, sachets, or craft into tablets and capsules to harvest the benefits you desire.

Safety Precautions: Avoid if suffering from depression, before and after surgery, with alcohol, and with sedatives.

LEMON BALM

(Melissa officinalis)

With the reputation of being able to lift the spirit and heal the heart, lemon balm was the ultimate "youth elixir." Being one of the key ingredients in cordials, a soft, diluted drink consumed during medieval times, this herb was very popular among royalty. The Prince of Gamogan, a county in Wales, used to drink lemon balm tea every day and actually lived for 108 years!

I don't know whether it will help us all live to be well past 100, but I can surely attest to lemon balm's amazing medicinal properties. I use it as a tonic for relieving aching flu symptoms, and it always manages to boost my spirits.

Native to: Europe, Northern Africa, Western Asia

Description: If you have lemon balm in your herbal garden, then you know how this lovely aromatic plant is adored by the bees. Once you experience its calming properties yourself, you will enjoy it just as much. From providing a sense of relaxation when you're feeling down, to relieving cold sores, to helping you restore your overactive thyroid function, this fragrant herb will definitely find its purpose in your home apothecary.

Main Components: Flavonoids, volatile oil, tannins, polyphenols, triterpenes

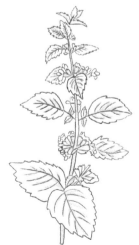

Medicinal Actions:
Relaxant
Carminative
Nerve Tonic
Antispasmodic
Antiviral, Especially for Herpes
Hormonal Herb

Main Uses:
Treats Overactive Thyroid
Relieves Cold Sores
Relieves Anxiety
Reduces Panic and Nervousness
Relieves Flu Symptoms
Treats Insect Stings

Parts Used: The aerial parts (the parts that grow above ground

Practical use: A very popular tincture, infusion, essential oil juice, lotion, or ointment, when needed.

Safety Precautions: Generally safe for everyone, but avoid i suffering from thyroid disease, as lemon balm is known to change the thyroid functioning.

LICORICE
(Glycyrrhiza glabra)

Did you know that licorice's main compound, glycyrrhizic acid, is 50 times sweeter than sugar? That is why if you look up 'candy in a thesaurus, you'll find it synonymous with licorice. Apart from its sugary taste, the root of this plant is one powerful herba medicine. In fact, a two-year study found that licorice extract is more effective for treating GERD (Gastroesophageal Reflux Disease) than conventional antacids (Setright, 2017).

My husband suffers from heartburn, so wherever he eats foods that upset his stomach, like orange juice or tomatoes, I prepare him a tincture which he consumes an hour after the meal. It feels very satisfying when all of his symptoms mysteriously disappear.

Native to: Europe, Southwest Asia

Description: Licorice root is one of the most effective herbal remedies. It is jam-packed with powerful anti-inflammatory properties, but it is also a powerful anti-arthritic herb. It supports the treatment of many conditions, from heartburn and arthritis to canker sores. It also serves as a gentle laxative to help battle constipation. In addition, licorice stimulates the adrenal glands. With all these uses, you don't need to feel guilty about picking up some licorice from the candy store again.

Main Components: Isoflavones, phytosterols, triterpene saponins, polysaccharides

Medicinal Actions:
Anti-inflammatory
Demulcent
Mild Laxative

Adrenal Agent
Anti-arthritic

Main Uses:
Treats Inflammatory Digestive Conditions
Treats Addison's Disease and Other Adrenal Issues
Relieves Arthritic Symptoms
Treats Menopausal Symptoms
Helps with Inflamed Joints
Soothes Inflamed Eyes

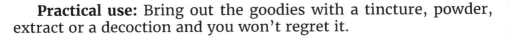

Parts Used: The root

Practical use: Bring out the goodies with a tincture, powder, extract or a decoction and you won't regret it.

Safety Precautions: Avoid during pregnancy as significant amounts of licorice increase the risk of early delivery. Also, avoid if suffering from high blood pressure, if you have hypertonia (a muscle condition), kidney problems, or you are taking Warfarin.

MILK THISTLE
(Silybum marianum)

The medicinal use of milk thistle can be traced back to the first century; and in Roman times, herbalists referred to this plant as the "carrier of bile" or the plant that could cleanse the internal fluids. Now a popular liver remedy in Western herbal medicine, many studies have backed up the efficacy of milk thistle (Mulrow et al., 2000).

My dear college friend made a life-threatening mistake when camping in Germany as a student. She and her boyfriend consumed death cap mushrooms thinking they were edible. Fortunately, just as their friend was about to put the grilled shroom in his mouth, he noticed that something was odd. He put two and two together and realized that the mushrooms they had just been grilling were incredibly deadly. They immediately went to the hospital and, two hours later, they received a medication with silymarin as a base. Silymarin is the extract from the seeds of milk thistle, and it protects the liver. It prevents highly toxic compounds from causing permanent damage to the liver and kidneys.

Native to: The Mediterranean

Description: Milk thistle can be found throughout Europe and now also commonly occurs in California. It is a spiny plant, with pink flowers, that thrives in sunny and open areas. It is mainly used for treating liver conditions, especially when the cells need to be renewed. It is a powerful remedy for hepatitis but is also perfect when the liver is under stress, such as during chemotherapy. As the name suggests, milk thistle also induces breast milk production.

Main Components: Flavonolignans, polyacetylenes, bitters

Medicinal Actions:
Liver Protective
Anti-allergenic
Chemoprotective
Anticancerous

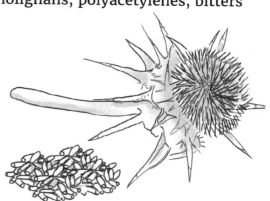

Main Uses:
Treats Liver Conditions
Treats Jaundice and Hepatitis
Supports Liver Function During Chemotherapy
Increases Breast Milk Production
Relieves Symptoms of Allergic Rhinitis

Parts Used: The flower heads and seeds

Practical use: A traditional herb which is frequently used in tinctures, decoctions, tablets, and capsules. And it's easy to imagine why, what with all its uses.

Safety Precautions: Avoid during pregnancy. Use only in appropriate doses, as a large amount of milk thistle can cause bloating, gas, nausea, and upset stomach. Avoid with hormone-sensitive conditions such as endometriosis or fibroid cancer, as milk thistle extract mimics estrogen.

NETTLE
(Urtica dioica)

Derived from the word "needle" and translated from Latin as "burn," this herb can inflict painful stings, as many people already know. But, aside from its sting, nettle can also give great healing to its users. It has various health benefits, but nettle's most recognized clinical action is its protection against benign prostatic hyperplasia (Ghorbanibirgani, 2013).

When I was pregnant with my daughter, I had severe iron deficiency. My OB told me that I would never be able to retrieve the normal iron levels with just herbs, and not stronger medications; I managed to prove him wrong. Among other herbal supplements, my main iron booster was my yummy nettle-leaf soup.

Native to: Temperate regions all over the world

Description: If you haven't felt a nettle's sting, then it is clear you are not spending enough time in nature. Leave the comfort of your home! Stinging nettle leaves have a long history of being quite the healer. This plant's anti-inflammatory and anti-allergenic compounds offer powerful protection from fever, arthritis, and anemia. Nettle is a cleansing and detoxifying herb that everyone should have in the herbal home apothecary. It is sought after, not only for its leaves, but also for its roots, which have just as many beneficial medical compounds trapped inside them.

Main Components: Amines, flavonoids, minerals, glucoquinone; phenols and sterols (root only)

Medicinal Actions:
Anti-inflammatory
Diuretic
Astringent
Anti-allergenic
Tonic
Prevents Hemorrhaging

Main Uses:
Increases Urine Production
Stops Bleeding from Wounds
Treats Nosebleeds
Treats Asthma and Hay Fever
Protects Liver Function
Relieves   Arthritic
Symptoms
Treats   Enlarged
Prostate Symptoms (the
root)

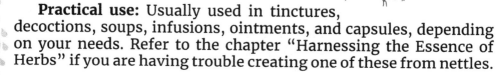

Parts Used: The leaves and root

Practical use: Usually used in tinctures, decoctions, soups, infusions, ointments, and capsules, depending on your needs. Refer to the chapter "Harnessing the Essence of Herbs" if you are having trouble creating one of these from nettles.

Safety Precautions: Avoid during pregnancy, as nettle can cause uterine contractions. Also, keep in mind that medication for diabetes interacts with nettle, as the plant also has glucose-lowering properties.

PEPPERMINT
(Mentha x piperita)

Just how old a cure is peppermint? History tells us that dried leaves were discovered in Egyptian pyramids. Clearly, Egyptian royalty thought peppermint wasn't only great for life, but for the afterlife as well. It is now 3000 years later, and we still depend on this powerful and fragrant herb for many conditions. Large clinical studies confirm that peppermint is an invaluable cure for treating irritable bowel syndrome (Chumpitazi et al., 2018).

After my C-section with my daughter, I struggled with bloating and gas, a common side effect from the abdominal operation. Peppermint tea and essential oil are packed with so many therapeutic properties that I was able to eat solids much sooner than I had anticipated.

Native to: Europe, North America, Asia

Description: Peppermint is more than the aromatic in your mojito. It is a powerful herbal medicine that carries with it a strong therapeutic effect. Rich in volatile oils and acting as an antibacterial, peppermint has a cooling effect on inflamed skin. It is also a powerful antiseptic. Its forte is treating digestive issues and giving pain relief, especially in the abdominal area. When peppermint essential oil is rubbed on the temples, it can also alleviate headache symptoms.

Main Components: Volatile oil, phenolic acids, flavonoids, triterpenes

Medicinal Actions:
Antiseptic
Antibacterial
Antispasmodic
Analgesic
Carminative
Antimicrobial
Stimulates Sweating

Main Uses:
Relieves Bloating, Gas, and Colic
Treats Digestive and Bowel Issues
Relaxes the Gut Muscles
Reduces Skin Sensitivity
Treats Eczema
Relieves Nausea
Soothes the Colon
Relieves Diarrhea
Relieves Pain (Especially Abdominal Pain and Headaches)

Parts Used: The aerial parts (that grow above the ground)

Practical use: A world-renowned herb which I use frequently when eating foods that produce gas, like legumes. Fine as infusions, teas, essential oils, ointments, and capsules. Keep in mind that this herb has many other use similar to the ones mentioned above.

Safety Precautions: Peppermint is generally safe for everyone However, those suffering from diarrhea should avoid peppermint as the herb can cause unpleasant anal burning. Peppermint also relaxes esophageal sphincters, which can make heartburn and GERD worse.

ROSEMARY
(Salvia rosmarinus)

With a ton of folklore uses and even more medicinal purposes rosemary deserves a special place in your herbal kit. Its main benefit is memory improvement, which is why many student. (especially in the Mediterranean) used to burn rosemary sprig when studying for exams.

My relationship with rosemary started in the kitchen but soon found a much better use for this natural and aromatic herb My rosemary tincture has guided me through many stressfu situations. When I feel the pressure piling up, I release steam by mixing 40 drops of rosemary extract with a glass of water Whether I am on a time crunch, trying to get work done for a project, or simply trying to finish my chores, rosemary is great for circulating blood to my head. It also lifts my spirits.

Native to: The Mediterranean

Description: Though it is one of the most used herbs in the world, rosemary does more than just enhance your culinary delicacies; it improves your health as well. Rosemary makes a warming tonic that soothes the nerves, promotes healthy blood flow, stimulates the adrenal glands, and uplifts the mood. It helps battle stress and mild depression, can ease rheumatic muscles and increases concentration. It is perfect for circulation, especially for people with low blood pressure.

Main Components: Volatile oil, tannins, rosmarinic acid, flavonoids, diterpenes

Medicinal Actions:
Anti-inflammatory
Stimulant
Nervine

Tonic
Antioxidant
Astringent

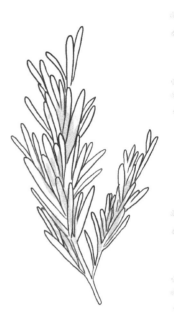

Main Uses:
Improves Concentration and Memory
Relaxes the Nerves
Relieves Stress and Tension
Raises Blood Pressure
Supports Circulation
Relieves Mild Symptoms of Depression
Relieves Headaches
Supports Hair Growth
Relieves Aching Muscles

Parts Used: The leaves

Practical use: Prepare it as a tincture, essential oil or an infusion, and it won't disappoint.

Safety Precautions: Safe if eaten, but should be avoided during pregnancy. Consume in appropriate doses as a high amount of rosemary causes kidney damage and stomach irritation. Avoid if you are allergic to aspirin.

SAGE
(Salvia officinalis)

Sage was a crucial part of the ancient Roman pharmacopeia. Romans used it frequently to support the digestion process after consuming fatty cuts of meat, popular at that time. Today, sage is often used as a preservative for meat, but that is not why this herb has found its way onto this list. Sage has a vast array of medicinal properties; the greatest of which is its antiseptic character. Hildegard of Bingen, a German Benedictine abbess, visionary, prophet, and herbalist who lived just over 900 years ago, famously said, "Why should a man die whilst sage grows in his garden."

A few months back, we were visiting some friends who had just moved to their farmhouse. The property was full of animals, had beautiful, lush gardens, and insects buzzing from flower to flower. While there, my daughter received a strange sting on her hand, that wasn't from a bee or a mosquito; unfortunately, my herbal kit was nowhere to be found. I looked around my friend's garden and saw sage among the herbs. I picked a few leaves and started rubbing them onto the sting site. Five minutes later the irritation was gone!

Native to: The Mediterranean

Description: As the meaning of its botanical name suggests (*salvere*; to be saved), sage does not only do wonders for our pork or our holiday meals, it also transforms our health. It is a powerful antiseptic, and effective in regulating hormonal activity. It is particularly helpful for hot flashes. Sage is a must–have herb for women in their 50s. There is also strong support for sage's beneficial effect on our nerves, but one of the most popular uses today is as a remedy for sore throats.

Main Components: Essential oil, tannins, diterpenes, phenolic compounds, triterpenes

Medicinal Actions:
Astringent
Estrogenic
Antiseptic

Nerve Tonic

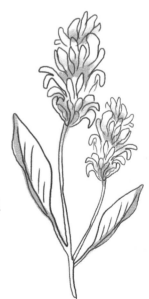

Main Uses:
Sore Throat Gargles
Digestive Tonic
Relieves Menopausal Symptoms
Supports Regular and Normal Menstrual Cycle
Lowers Blood Fat Levels
Decreases Depression Symptoms
Enhances Memory
Relieves Bites and Stings

Parts Used: The leaves

Practical use: Prepare as a tincture, infusion, or tea.

Safety Precautions: Not recommended during pregnancy, as it contains thujone, a chemical that induces the menstrual cycle. Sage also lowers blood sugar and can interact with medication for diabetes. It can also interact with seizure drugs.

ST. JOHN'S WORT
(Hypericum perforatum)

St. John's Wort has recently been revived as an herbal remedy, in all its medieval glory! Although we can no longer say that it protects us from evil influences, a belief of many medieval people, this yellow summer flower brings dozens of medicinal uses to your home apothecary.

My dear friend, who was suffering from postpartum depression, took a St. John's Wort tincture a couple of times a day and was able to overcome her mental hardships quickly. During the Middle Ages, this flower was believed to cure insanity and, though people no longer suffer from "general insanity," this herb is still extremely useful for treating mental exhaustion.

Native to: Temperate Regions Throughout the World

Description: These summer yellow flowers not only look good in your vase, but they can also do wonders for your mental well-being. Known as one of the most powerful herbal antidepressants, St. John's Wort is a nerve tonic that restores and keeps our mood in check. Still, that's not the only way we benefit from these lovely flowers. St. John's Wort is also excellent for repairing tissue, and its oil is one of the most effective alternative medicines for post-surgery recovery.

Main Components: Flavonoids, phloroglucinols, polycyclic diones

Medicinal Actions:
Antidepressant
Anti-inflammatory
Anxiolytic

Antiviral
Tissue Repair

Main Uses:
Treats Depression Symptoms
Calms the Nerves

Lowers Anxiety
Promotes Recovery After Surgeries
Heals Wounds and Burns
Improves Lowered Mood During Menopause

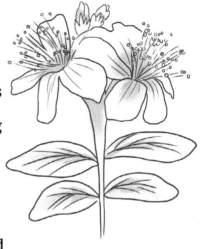

Parts Used: The flowering tops

Practical use: This is one of the herbs best used fresh, to make tinctures, infusions, infused oils, and creams.

Safety Precautions: Not recommended during pregnancy as some studies suggest it causes birth defects. Also not recommended during breastfeeding as it can cause colic and drowsiness in infants.

TURMERIC
(Curcuma longa)

This Indian cuisine staple offers more than a bit of spice or a dash of yellow color to your meals. It is one of the most powerful and oldest medicinal foods in existence. Every herbal healer should keep a hefty supply of turmeric around. Records of turmeric's use for medicinal purposes date from more than 4,000 years ago.

Although the therapeutic actions of this golden spice started gaining attention only a few decades ago, every alternative medicine aficionado will confirm that having turmeric in your home apothecary is a must. And I am here to attest to its incredible anti-inflammatory properties. I have Hashimoto's disease, which is an autoimmune illness of the thyroid, and taking my turmeric tincture with water is what keeps the paths of inflammation clear.

Native to: India, Southeast Asia

Description: This most valuable remedy in Indian culture has spread throughout the world in recent decades, and for good reason! Turmeric is a powerful medicinal agent that can support and improve our health in many different ways. It has shown benefits, from fighting inflammation to lowering cholesterol (Hewlings & Kalman, 2017). It is a key ingredient in beating chronic health issues. The yummy golden powder and its main constituent, curcumin, have unparalleled medicinal use.

Main Components: Curcumin, resin, volatile oil, bitters

Medicinal Actions:
Anti-inflammatory
Antimicrobial
Lowers Cholesterol
Antiplatelet

Main Uses:
Fights Inflammation
Relieves Allergies
Treats Autoimmune Diseases
Supplement for Dementia, Diabetes, and Cancer
Lowers Cholesterol Levels
Keeps the Blood Thin
Protects the Stomach and Liver by Increasing Bile Production
Beneficial for Gastritis
Assists with Eczema, when Applied to the Skin

Parts Used: The rhizome (broken, boiled, and then dried)

Practical use: Turmeric is used as a tincture, powder, and decoction. I often personally use the powdered form in my soups. I use it when cooking as it gives that beautiful golden color to white meat and vegetables. It also smells divine!

Safety Precautions: Generally safe, but not recommended for people suffering from gallbladder conditions. It also interacts with anticoagulant medications.

VERVAIN

(Verbena officinalis)

Vervain is one of the most popular "magical" herbs. But despite its contribution to witchcraft and ritual ceremonies, it has also left an incredible mark on the scientific world and on the history of herbal medicine.

When the holiday season rolls over, I turn into a binge eater. Although it doesn't show on my body, as I run off most of my calories, trust me when I tell you that I can eat a lot. Last Christmas, there were so many leftovers (I not only binge eat, but binge cook as well) that I thought swallowing them up was the best way to prevent my hard work from going to waste. A couple of hours later, my tummy ached like a toddler's after eating too many candies. A vervain infusion did the trick and helped relieve all the pressure in my stomach. Vervain helps the digestive system absorb food quickly and restores gut balance!

Native to: Southern Europe

Description: Acting as a cure for nearly every ailment throughout the centuries, vervain is a versatile herb with many medicinal properties. Its uses stretch from stimulating the womb, to supporting digestion and dealing with headaches. It also does wonders for our nervous system. It is safe to say that, whatever health issue you're dealing with, there is certainly some benefit that vervain can bring your way. If none of these reasons is enough to convince you to add vervain to your herb garden, consider that it can also be used as toothpaste! Powdered vervain rubbed on the teeth and gums can keep them clean and protected.

Main Components: Flavonoids, alkaloids, bitter iridoids, volatile oil, triterpenes

Medicinal Actions:
Mild Antidepressant
Nervine
Tonic

Main Uses:
Deals with Digestive Issues
Relieves Nervous Tension
Good for Reducing Depression Symptoms

Tonic for Chronic Illnesses
Relieves Headaches and Migraines
Relieves Premenstrual Syndrome

Parts Used: The aerial parts (that grow above ground)

Practical use: This herb is commonly prepared as a tincture, infusion, and powder.

Safety Precautions: Generally recognized as safe, but not recommended during pregnancy.

YARROW
(Achillea millefolium)

Did you know that Achilles, a hero of the Trojan War in Greek mythology, shares his name with this white flower? In fact, it is thought that these white flowers helped this Greek legend heal his wounds on the battlefield. Whether Achilles was named after the herb, or the herb has gotten the name thanks to the way it helped heal him heal, is up for a debate. But what's certain is this: yarrow is a heavenly herb for healing.

When my husband cut his arm on one of our frequent outdoor adventures, I applied yarrow poultice onto the cut and wrapped it up tightly. When we got home, we were both surprised to see how very little blood there was. While that was my first experience of yarrow in action, I can definitely attest that Achilles was right – applying yarrow on wounds will keep them clean and stop blood flow.

Native to: Europe, North America, Western Asia

Description: With similar healing properties as chamomile, yarrow is another essential herb you should never be without. With tons of powerful constituents that bring incredible health benefits, it is no surprise this plant has a long-standing reputation among herbalists. Yarrow minimizes external and internal bleeding; it dilates the blood vessels, has antitumor properties, and it is also powerful in fighting against the common cold and flu by encouraging sweating and reducing the fever.

Main Components: Flavonoids, volatile oil, alkaloids,

sesquiterpene lactones, tannins, triterpenes, phytosterols

Medicinal Actions:
Bitter Tonic
Astringent
Anti-inflammatory
Antispasmodic
Mild Diuretic
Stops Bleeding

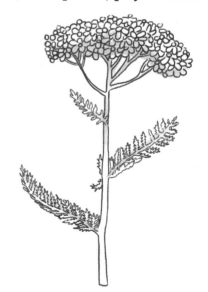

Main Uses:
Treats Wounds
Lowers Blood Pressure
Reduces Fever
Regulates Menstrual Flow
Decreases Cold and Flu Symptoms
Tones Varicose Veins
Helps with Digestive Infections

Parts Used: The aerial parts (that grow above ground)

Practical use: Great for tinctures, essential oils, and poultices. This herb may help you greatly with digestive issues, wound healing, depression, and anxiety, and fighting inflammation; it truly is nature's gift. Then again, which herb is not?

Safety Precautions: Avoid during pregnancy and when breastfeeding. Yarrow also slows blood clotting and shouldn't be taken with anticoagulant medications.

All the previously mentioned herbs are loaded with helpful constituents that provide powerful medicinal actions. The trick to squeezing the most out of them lies in using them correctly. After adding these rich and powerful ingredients to your herbal magic kit, it is time to take the next step. It is time to learn how to start your own medicinal garden and make sure that you are equipped with the right tools for extracting the active ingredients. If you are ready to lay the foundations of your home apothecary, jump to the next chapter!

Your
Own Medicine Garden
and Home Apothecary

ow that you know what medicinal herbs you should take advantage of to support your overall health, the time has come to think about setting up your own home apothecary. In the ideal scenario, your home apothecary is also accompanied by a lush herb garden – a place that will allow you to gather the needed herbs for your remedies in the most convenient way possible. Let's face it though, most of us live under conditions that are far from ideal. The lucky ones who have settled in far-flung rural corners, surrounded by acres of land, can exploit and experiment with various plants, as they see fit. But should that mean that those living in small apartments are doomed never to try their hand at growing herbs? Definitely not!

Not all herbs demand large spaces or constant sunlight. Some actually thrive in a windowsill garden. So, whether you grow them next to a window, in a corner in your kitchen, on your balcony, or in a small backyard, anyone can hop onto the herb-growing bandwagon.

If you don't already have a medicinal herb garden, there are a few factors to consider before getting started:

The Place – Growing indoors, outdoors, or under a cover (such as inside a greenhouse) will all require slightly different approaches.

If you plan on cultivating the herbs in your

backyard, choose hardy plants with roots that can penetrate deeply, and with lush foliage that will provide a plentiful harvest. If the plants aren't hardy, you should think about moving them someplace sheltered.

If planting indoors, choose a hanging basket, container, window box, or a small flowerpot for the herbs to do their magic. Extra precaution is needed when growing indoors, as herbs can dry out or outgrow their pots. If they are kept in conditions that are less than ideal, then the possibility of these events becomes all-the-more likely. Transplant to larger containers, when needed, to prevent the plants from becoming pot bound. Aloe vera, basil, calendula, chamomile, lavender, lemon balm, rosemary, sage, St. John's wort, thyme, and yarrow all thrive indoors.

If you have a greenhouse, then you have a few more options. You can tweak the growing conditions and adjust the temperature and humidity as you see fit, so it will be possible to grow a range of exotic and more "needy" herbs.

The Sun Exposure – Whether indoors or outdoors, there is one thing that all herbs require: proper sun exposure. Medicinal herbs thrive in sunny areas, so make sure to provide a proper place to nourish your sweet little plants. Inside, place the containers near the windows or someplace where they can get plenty of natural light. Outside, find sunny corners and avoid spots where larger plants, trees, or buildings cast shadows during the day.

The Soil – Most herbs need well-drained soil. If growing indoors, make sure to buy potting soil and never fill the containers with outdoor soil. Firstly, that soil is a lot heavier and, more importantly, it can contain bacteria and diseases that can eventually kill your indoor herbs.

If growing outdoors, make sure to analyze the soil first and establish that it is a healthy growing medium. Take handfuls of soil, gathered from different spots in the garden, and check them with a soil test kit, which is available from most gardening stores. Check the soil pH and see what kind of compost will be best to enrich the soil. Most medicinal plants require a pH of 6.3–6.8.

Once you take care of the essentials, you should then decide whether to cultivate from seed or buy your medicinal plants from an herb nursery. If choosing the latter, pay attention that you buy standard medicinal plants, as many herbs are improved and sold mainly for ornamental purposes.

Proper Maintenance – Immediately after planting, you should give your plants and seeds enough water to kickstart healthy growth. After that, it is probably wise to water your herbs only once or twice a week, rather than water them every single day. Remember, the point is not to overwater, as the medicinal actions are the greatest when the conditions are drier.

When it comes to feeding the herbs, keep in mind that giving mulch or other fertilizers to your medicinal plants may lower their potency and therapeutic properties. However, that doesn't mean that you shouldn't treat the soil before planting. The soil must be nutritious enough to provide a healthy environment for the herbs.

If your plants are diseased or infected, separate them from the healthy ones, and treat with organic cures only. A good solution may be to soak garlic in water and then spray it over the plants in order to repel pests.

Harvesting and Processing

Whether you have your own garden or are an outdoor aficionado like me, and love the thrill of looking for herbs in the wild, proper harvesting and processing are crucial for the quality and intensity of the medicinal actions of the plants.

Harvesting from the Wild

The wild offers an abundance of free medicinal herbs. Harvesting herbs in the wild makes you feel truly connected with nature and with the inner herbal-healing instincts that you possess! But what I love most about this harvesting method is that wild-grown herbs are more concentrated than those found in your home garden. That means that wild medicinal plants will have a more powerful effect on your health than the herbs growing in containers in your home. However, as appealing as this sounds, there are quite a few concerns you need to pay attention to:

Identification – I cannot stress this enough! Proper identification is essential. Improper identification can possibly be life-threatening. It's easy to mistake a harmful wild plant for some medicinal herb. For instance, poisonous foxglove leaves are often mistaken for comfrey. So, before you head out to the great, wild woods with your rucksack in tow, make sure you know your herbs well, as misidentification can easily lead to serious problems.

The Site – You may be tempted to harvest nettles that grow by the road, but I strongly suggest you rethink that urge. Plants growing near roadsides, factories, or even fields where the crop might be sprayed with pesticides, should most certainly be avoided. Instead, try to go deep in nature, far from sources of pollution or other areas where plants may be in contact with artificial materials.

Other Ecological Factors – Never harvest more plants than you plan to use. In addition, do not uproot wild herbs; instead, make a clean cut with a sharp knife or scissors. Keep in mind that bark shouldn't be collected from the wild, as stripping this layer from the tree can put the whole plant at risk.

When harvesting in the wild, place the cut herbs inside a nylon sack and make sure not to pack them too tightly together.

Harvesting from Your Garden

If you're cultivating your own garden, then you have medicinal herbs always at your fingertips. All you have to do is simply gather what you need. But as simple as it sounds, there is actually more to harvesting herbs than just cutting them with a pair of scissors. It must be done with gentle, tender care, as being too rough with these precious herbs may put the entire plant's chance of survival at risk.

Here are the four steps to harvesting properly from one's garden:

#1 Gather the Right Equipment – The most important part of harvesting herbs is to do so with a clean cut. It is also vital that you avoid crushing the herbs you have cut. I recommend a pair of sharp scissors and an open tray or basket.

#2 Harvest at the Right Time – It goes without saying that you should harvest your plants at peak maturity to ensure the highest concentration of beneficial compounds. As a general rule, herb plants gain strength towards the time of flowering; many are strong enough to use all season, but they are strongest just before flowering. Leaves are best harvested just before budding. Flowers are best harvested when most are still in the bud stage, but a few have opened. If you wait, the flowers will be pollinated, and their properties then diminish rapidly, sometimes in only a few days. At this stage, the plant puts all its energy into developing seeds. Fruits and berries can be harvested when they become ripe, and the root can be collected in autumn, or when the plant starts drawing the nutrients from the aerial parts into the ground parts.

#3 Harvest the Right Parts – Keep in mind that different parts of the plant have different medicinal actions. Do your due diligence before harvesting, to make sure that the collected herbs will address your condition properly.

#4 Harvest the Right Amount – Never gather more than you need, period. If you're not about to process, or not planning to use the herbs immediately after harvesting, do not collect as many. If using for salads or cooking, the herbs are best consumed right after harvesting. If making remedies, it is recommended that you process them as soon as possible.

Preserving the Harvested Herbs

Did you know that aromatic herbs lose the majority of their powerful volatile oils only a few hours after being harvested? That's why processing the harvested herbs at a low temperature, and as quickly as possible, is crucial in order to prevent the medicinal compounds from deteriorating rapidly.

There are many ways in which you can process the herbs to preserve their active constituents, but the easiest and simplest of all is by letting them dry naturally in the air, or by popping them into a cool oven to dry for a bit of time.

Stems and Leaves

When harvesting stems, make sure to separate the flowers and large leaves from the bunch, as they should each be processed in a slightly different way.

The stems and smaller leaves should be gathered in a bunch of eight to ten. Then it is important to secure with them with some strand – not too tightly, as there should be room for air circulation between the stems and leaves. Hang them upside down in a dark and warm place that is not too hot and has good ventilation. If the air is very humid, use artificial heat like your oven or a dehydrator for the drying process. Check in on the herbs daily, and when the stems and leaves become brittle, but not so dry that they crumble, they're ready. Grab a tray or a piece of newspaper and rub the stems with both your hands to separate the small leaves.

Flowers

For large flowers, separate them immediately after harvesting, and inspect well to remove any insects. Line a tray with a piece of absorbent paper and arrange the flowers in a single layer on the tray. Then place the tray in a warm, dark, well-ventilated spot.

Smaller flowers can be harvested while still attached to the stalk and then hung in bunches, just like stems. With flowers, I suggest putting them in a paper bag first and then securing them with a strand.

If you plan to use only the petals, and not the whole flower head, be sure to remove the petals before storing; then discard the heads.

Berries and Fruit

Fruits and berries should be harvested when they reach peak ripeness, not only because they are the most effective at that stage, but also because they may not dry properly if overripe.

Arrange them on a tray lined with absorbent paper, and pop inside a warmed oven. The oven should not be on – just warm. Do not close the oven door. Instead, crack it open, and let the fruits sit for about four hours. Then, move the tray to a warm and dimly lit place. Check the berries and fruits daily, turning them over occasionally, until they have dried out fully.

Roots, Rhizomes, and Bulbs

After harvesting the plants' underground parts, you should wash them thoroughly to get rid of the dirt. Dry them with some paper towels. Chop the roots or bulbs finely; they will dry faster if small, and most become rock hard after drying. If there are any damaged parts, discard them.

Just as with the berries, place the chopped roots onto a tray lined with absorbent paper, place in a warmed oven with the door open, and allow to sit for a couple of hours. Then move the tray to a dark and warm area, and keep it there until the roots are completely dried.

Seeds

Gather the seed heads into small bunches, tie them together, and hang them upside down in a warm, dark, well-ventilated place. If the seeds are tiny, you can place the heads in a paper bag before tying them together. When dried, gently shake them inside the bag, to help free the seeds from the heads.

Bark

As I've mentioned before, gathering bark from the wild is not a good idea as a plant that loses its bark will die. However, if you already have your own medicinal shrubs, you can harvest the beneficial bark from outlying branches, with extra care and love. Later, you can prune back those areas with minimal damage done to the plant.

Chop the bark up finely, arrange on a tray, and place in a dark and warm area to dry in the air.

Gel and Sap

Harvest gel and sap with care and only while wearing gloves, as the milky juices can often be corrosive. You can collect these liquids by squeezing the stems over a bowl. If gathering aloe vera gel, you can do it by cutting the leaves lengthwise and then peeling the edges off.

Gel and sap do not need to be processed, as they already are in their medicinal forms.

Storing the Herbs

If not stored properly, your herbs will not last. Be sure they are completely crisp dry before storing, as the slightest bit of moisture will allow mold to grow. Once they are dried, you can place them in sterilized, opaque glass containers with air-tight lids. Alternatively, you can choose a more inexpensive option and store them in new and unused brown paper bags. Be cautious when using the paper bag method of storage because your herbs will require an especially dark and dry place for storage. Keep in mind that the lifespan of your brown-bagged herbs is much shorter. Air-tight storage is much more effective; herbs in air-tight jars can last a full year after harvesting, while those in brown bags only last about six months.

For gel and sap, if not using right away, you can simply pour the liquid into an ice cube tray and freeze for prolonged lifespan and convenient use.

Important: Never store your herbs in plastic or metal containers, regardless of their quality. Metal and plastic can ooze chemicals that may contaminate the herbs.

With your apothecary now full of dried herbs, let's learn how to use them and extract the trapped goodies inside, so you can address your health issues the natural way.

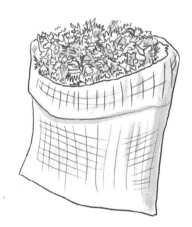

Harnessing the Essence of Herbs

ven the most well-stocked home apothecary will not be beneficial if you fail to extract the medicinal properties out of the herbs correctly. Each of the plants mentioned in this book comes with valuable constituents, which are trapped in different parts of the plant. To become a real herbalist, it is your job to understand which parts provide the most important medicinal actions, and more importantly, how to extract the active components and turn them into a readily available medicine.

Nothing is better than munching on fresh herbs! However, this is inconvenient with modern life, doesn't work well with barks and doesn't preserve the herbs for the cold season. The following methods of extraction, chosen with each specific herb in mind, allow you to access everything potent in the plant all year round. This is something you cannot possibly achieve while simply munching on the leaves.

There are many different extraction methods: these include basic infusions, soaking in alcohol, extracting powders, and making topical applications. All of these methods will be covered in this herbal book. Herbal extracts come in the form of liquids, creams, powders, and oils, all of which contain substances that can address different health issues.

It may sound like a daunting task at this point but

you don't necessarily need extensive herbal knowledge or herbal family roots to harness the essence of the medicinal plants you've chosen to grow. All you need is the right guidance and clear instructions to follow, which are covered in this next chapter. So, hop on this herbal train and get ready for the magical act of whipping up herbal potions, creams, tinctures, and all sorts of mixtures that will do wonders for your health.

Infusions

As the name suggests, infusion is a process in which the dried herbs are steeped in an absorbing liquid, water being the easiest one to use. The process is like making tea. Although tea is an infusion, not all infusions are tea. Often, it's alcohol that is used as the liquid to make a tincture, or oil that is destined for a salve. This is the simplest and most straightforward way to use the aerial parts of the plant for medicine. The only difference between brewing a tea for pleasure and one for medicinal purposes, is strength. A medicinal infusion is stronger, usually because of a longer steeping time, but sometimes also because of the amount of herb used. Tea is a more neutral and mellow drink, which is why it is widely enjoyed; infusions aren't normally so tasty.

To make a hot water infusion, normally just called an infusion, you will need:

- A Kettle

- A Tea Strainer

- A Cup with a Lid

- Your Herbs of Choice

- Hot Water

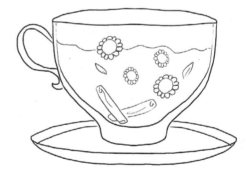

How to infuse:

1. Boil some water in a kettle.

2. Place about a teaspoon of the preferred dried herb in a strainer.

3. Place the strainer inside the cup and pour the boiling water over the top of the herbs.

4. Cover the cup with a lid and let it steep for seven to ten minutes before removing the lid.

5. Remove the strainer with the herbs, catching the last precious drips of medicine.

6. Sweeten with some honey, if desired, and enjoy warm or cold.

Alternatively, you can perform an infusion in a pot. You will need:

– A Kettle

– A Pot with a Lid

– A Cup

– Hot Water

– Herbs of Your Choice

– A Mesh Strainer

How to infuse in a pot:

1. Boil some water in the kettle and pour two cups of the boiling water inside the pot.

2. Add about 20 g (0.7 oz) of dried herbs and place the lid atop the pot.

3. Let sit for ten minutes.

4. Place the mesh strainer over the cup and strain the infusion into the cup.

5. Enjoy!

The key to making an infusion is to <u>cover the cup while steeping</u>. Most medicinal actions in the herbs are due to the presence of volatile oil, which can quickly be dispersed into the air if you're steeping without a lid.

Tip: To make herbal tea, the process is pretty much the same. Cut down the steeping time to five minutes, so that the tea isn't quite so potent. That's it!

<u>Dosage</u>: A standard dosage is to take about 3 cups of infusion per day. Of course, this varies from herb to herb, as some have a stronger taste and effect, while others can be quite refreshing (e.g., yarrow vs. chamomile). If the herb is quite intense and you decide to take a large dose, the infusion can end up having a negative effect.

<u>*Storage:*</u> Infused beverages can be stored in a covered pot, bowl, or jug in the fridge, for up to 24 hours.

Cold Infusions

For some conditions, you may need to extract the herbs using a cold infusion. Some active constituents can be destroyed when introduced to heat; the process of infusing herbs in cold water is called cold infusion.

For a cold infusion, you will need:

- A Bowl
- A Fine-Mesh Strainer
- A Jug
- Water
- Herbs

Performing a cold infusion:

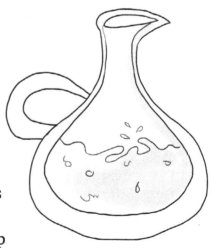

1. Combine the herbs and water in a clean bowl. For 25–30 g (about 1 oz) of herbs, I recommend 2 cups of water.

2. Let the mixture steep overnight.

3. Place the fine-mesh strainer over the jug and pour the contents of the bowl through the strainer and into the jug.

4. Consume a cold infusion as you would consume a hot water infusion or a decoction.

Storage: Cover and place in the fridge; consume within the next 48 hours.

Decoctions

Not all parts of the plants can be easily infused. If you need to extract bark, roots, or berries, you will need a slightly stronger approach. Decoctions are a slightly more complex trick up an herbalist's sleeve but do not worry, you can make them too. Decoction is a process of extraction in which the herbs are simmered in boiling water.

In Chinese medicine, decoctions are the preferred method of extraction. Chinese herbalists make especially concentrated decoctions by adding many different herbs to the potion or simmering for a long time, until the liquid is reduced to less than a cup.

Decoctions are mainly used for drinking, but they are also effective if applied externally, such as for washes.

To make a decoction, you will need:

- A Saucepan
- A Jug
- A Mesh Strainer
- Herbs
- Water
- A Stove

How to make a decoction:

1. Place the herbs inside the saucepan. For a daily dosage, add about 20 g (0.7 oz) of dried herbs or 40 g (1.4 oz) of fresh ones. If using a mixture of herbs, go with 40 g (1.7 oz) in total.

2. Cover the herbs with cold water (3 cups for a daily dosage) and place them over medium heat.

3. Bring the liquid to a boil, then lower the heat and let simmer for 20–30 minutes. The strained liquid should be reduced from 3 cups to 2 cups in volume.

4. Remove the saucepan from heat.

5. Place the mesh strainer over a jug and pour the liquid through the strainer.

6. Consume as needed.

If the mood strikes you, you can also add more delicate parts to the decoction. If you think you will benefit more if you add some flowers, leaves, or stems to the mix, place them inside the pot, just after you turn off the heat. That way, they will start to infuse as the mixture begins to cool.

Dosage: Just as with the infusion, the right dosage depends on the herbal intensity but, for most plants, a daily decoction of 2 cups will do the trick. You can take a decoction warm or cold.

Storage: Cooled, leftover decoction can be stored in a covered pot or jug and refrigerated for up to 48 hours.

Tinctures

Tinctures really pack a punch. Made by soaking herbs in alcohol, this extraction is probably the strongest method of all. Tinctures can be different strengths depending on the herb-to-alcohol ratio, and the strength of the alcohol used, among other factors. Alcohol is measured in terms of concentration (proof) and volume (liquid ounces, liters or milliliters), while herb content is measured in weight (grams or ounces).

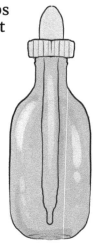

Tinctures are classified according to the ratio of herb to menstruum (solvent), with the menstruum being composed partly of alcohol, and partly of water. The aim, when making a tincture, is to end up with a final product that is at least 20% alcohol, so that the tincture is shelf stable. Most tinctures work well with vodka because that menstruum ratio is 40:60 (40 units of herb to 60 units of menstruum) or 50:50, and the active medicinal components are mostly water soluble. The alcohol concentration is high enough that the finished product is 20% (40-proof) or higher, ensuring that the tincture will be shelf stable.

If the herb being used is fresh, the juice and active components will be extracted out of the plant cells and will dilute the alcohol-water solvent. Thus, when making a tincture out of juicy leaves, for example, one must start with stronger alcohol, to allow for the extra dilution that will take place. Examples of these herbs are lemon balm and St. John's wort. When using a gum or resin, like myrrh, the alcohol needs to be near 95% (200-proof).

Tips on alcohol amount and strength

80 to 90 proof vodka (40-45% ethanol content). Fill 40% to 50% alcohol by volume.
· The usual percentage range for tinctures.
· Suitable for fresh herbs with low moisture and dried herbs.
· Suitable for extracting water-soluble active components.

Half 80 proof (40% ethanol) vodka & half 190 proof (95% ethanol) grain alcohol. Fill 67.5% to 70% alcohol by volume.
· Suitable for extracting those volatile aromatic components.
· Suitable for fresh and juicy herbs. Berries, aromatic roots, and lemon balm for example.
· The stronger alcohol concentration will extract the plant juices.

190 proof grain alcohol (95% ethanol content). Fill 85% to 95% alcohol by volume.
· Suitable for extracting the aromatic components and essential oils that don't dissolve easily.
· Suitable for diffusing gums and resins but not necessary for other plant parts.
· This alcohol strength will dehydrate your herbs if botanicals other than gums and resins are being tinctured.

Important: Never prepare tinctures with industrial alcohol, rubbing alcohol, or methyl alcohol!

If you still find this a bit daunting, after doing your research on the specific herbs you wish to use and asking your herbalist friends, the Facebook group "Herbalism For Beginners At Home – Medicinal Herbs and Herbalist Remedies" is a great place to ask for guidance.

Although most popular in Western herbal medicine, tinctures also have a long, traditional use. These preparations are very convenient to use, can be prepared with pretty much any herb and can be applied to treat a wide variety of health concerns.

To make a tincture yourself, you will need:

A Large Clean Jar with a Lid
A Muslin Bag (Nylon Mesh or Cheesecloth also Work Well)
A Large Pot (or Wine Press)
Small Dark Glass Bottles
A Funnel
Vodka
Preferred Herbs

How to create a tincture:
1. Place the herbs in a clean and sterilized jar, and pour the vodka over them. If using fresh herbs, you can go with a 1:2 ratio, adding double the weight of alcohol to your fresh herbs. If using dried herbs, though, the suggested ratio is 1:5. You should pour five times the weight of vodka into the jar as you have herbs.

2. With more potent herbs, the ratio could be 1:10 or even 1:20. Do prior research on the specific herbs and ask your herbalist friends, in order to determine a suitable herb-to-vodka ratio. Put the lid on, and secure tightly. Shake the jar well for a couple of minutes, then place it in a warm and dark place. (You can speed up the making of tincture with warmth – around 38°C or 100°F.Leave it there for about 10–14 weeks, making sure to shake the jar for a minute or two every couple of days.

3. When the time for straining comes, place the clean muslin bag over the large pot or wine press. If using a wine press, simply press it strongly to extract the tincture. If straining over a regular pot, just pour the jar contents carefully

through the cloth, then bring the edges of the cloth together, trapping the herbs inside, and squeeze to extract well. Alternatively, you can do this with a regular mesh strainer.

4. Using a funnel, carefully transfer the strained liquid into the sterilized dark glass bottles. Seal tightly!

5. Although vodka is the alcohol of choice for most herbalists, you can also use rum, especially if you include bitter herbs. The taste of the rum can mellow out the non-pleasing herbal taste.

Dosage: The standard dose is to take about a teaspoon of tincture diluted in about 1 ½ tbsp of water or juice, two or three times a day, depending on the herbs used.

Storage: Store the sealed dark glass bottles in a dark and cool place. Properly stored tinctures will remain safe to use for up to two years.

Syrups

We grownups may be fine with drinking infusions and decoctions, but children are usually not big fans of these herbal remedies, especially if we're using unpalatable and bitter plants. And what better way to force them to take their medicine than with a sugary bribe? That's when syrups come to the rescue!

Syrups are made with equal amounts of infusion and honey or unrefined sugar. In addition to being sweet in taste, syrups also come with an added benefit; they bring an extra soothing action to the mix, which is why they are so effective for treating sore throats and coughs. Besides this, they are also jam-packed with sugar which is a natural preservative. This helps the infusion or decoction survive for months on the shelf.

The important thing to know about making syrups with infusions and decoctions is that the herbs must be infused for the maximum time for the maximum potency. If using an infusion, steep for a full 15 minutes, and if using a decoction, simmer for half an hour.

To make a syrup, you will need:

- A Saucepan
- A Wooden Spatula
- Dark Glass Bottles
- A Funnel
- Infusion or Decoction
- Honey or Refined Sugar
- A Stove

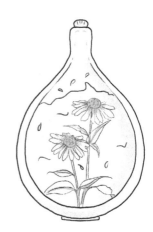

How to create a syrup:

1. Add about two cups of the prepared infusion or decoction into a saucepan.

2. Add the honey at this point – 500 g (17.6 oz) for 2 cups of infusion, or half the amount if only using 1 cup of infused liquid.

3. Stir over low heat, until the honey or sugar is fully mixed.

4. Turn off the heat and allow the saucepan to cool down.

5. Use a funnel and pour the syrup into dark, sterilized glass bottles.

6. Secure tightly and use the syrup as needed.

You can also make a syrup with a tincture. For this preparation, you will need:

- 500 g (17.6 oz) Honey or Unrefined Sugar
- 1 cup Water
- Tincture
- A Saucepan
- A Wooden Spatula

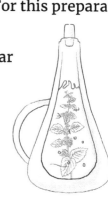

- A Jug

- A Funnel

- Dark Glass Bottles

- A Stove

To make a syrup with a tincture:

1. Combine the honey (or sugar) with the water in the saucepan.

2. Place over medium heat, and heat gently, stirring until the sugar or honey is dissolved.

3. Remove the saucepan from heat and allow the syrup to cool completely.

4. Place one part of your preferred tincture into a jug and add three parts of the syrup to it. If using ¼ cup of a tincture, add ¾ cup of the syrup.

5. Stir to combine and pour into your sterilized dark glass bottles with the help of a funnel.

6. Close and use the syrup as needed.

Dosage: Take about 1–2 teaspoons of the syrup, three times a day.

Storage: Store the dark glass bottles in a dark and cool place, and consume the syrup within the next six months.

Infused Oils

You may be familiar with this method for adding a bit of flavor to your dishes, but infusing herbs in oil can be quite beneficial for your health as well. By infusing the medicinal plants this way, you encourage their fat-soluble constituents to be released. In the process, you unlock compounds that you otherwise cannot extract.

There are two oil infusion methods: hot infusion, by simmering herbs in oil over gentle heat; and cold infusion, by letting the herbs naturally and gradually release their goodies at room temperature. Since the beneficial compounds in herbs can break down at temperatures of above 100°C (212°F), so cold infusion is the preferred method.

When making infused oils, no drops of water should get into the oil. This can support microbial growth and ruin the infusion. For this reason, it is preferable to use dried herbs in your infusions. However, if you wish to use fresh herbs (which give a stronger flavor), you should first rinse the herbs to clean them, then pat with paper towel and leave overnight to dry and wilt completely in the air, before adding them to the oil. Hot infusions keep for longer, but cold infusions can still be stored in the refrigerator for several months. If you notice any unusual smell to your infusion, it has possibly become contaminated with bacteria or mold and should be discarded.

Hot Infusion

Hot-infused oil can be used in many ways, from drizzling over meals for flavor, to applying by rubbing oil onto the skin for therapeutic massage and healing purposes. It can even be used as a secret ingredient in your ointments. You can use olive, sunflower, or any decent-quality vegetable oil for this purpose.

You will need:

- A Saucepan

- A Heat-Resistant Glass Bowl with a Lid

- A Wide-Mouthed Jug or Simple Pot

- A Muslin Bag or Cheesecloth

- A Dark Glass Bottle

- A Funnel

- Herbs

- Vegetable Oil

- A Stove

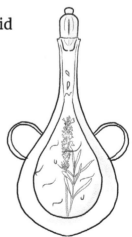

And here is how to do it:

1. Place about 1 cup (250 g or 8.8 oz) of dried herbs in a clean glass bowl.

2. Pour between 1¼ and 1½ C of oil over the herbs, and give the mixture a stir.

3. Fill the saucepan half way with water and place it over medium heat. Bring to a boil.

4. Place the glass bowl in the mouth of the saucepan, so that the base of the bowl is resting in the warm water. Cover the glass bowl with a lid, and allow to heat gently for at least a couple of hours. (Alternatively, you can use a double boiler for this.)

5. Keep the temperature of the oil between 38 and 60°C (100–140°F).

6. Remove the bowl from the heat and allow to cool until it is safe to handle.

7. Place the muslin bag over the wide-mouthed jug, tucking the middle of the cloth inside, while the sides remain over the jug, so there is no mess while pouring.

8. Pour the oil gently through the muslin bag. Bring the edges of the cloth together, trapping the herbs inside, and gently squeeze to extract the strained liquid into the jug.

9. With the help of a funnel, pour the strained oil into the previously sterilized bottle. Seal tightly and use as needed.

Cold Infusion

Cold infusion is a much slower process, but it is the preferred method because it preserves the active compounds and gives a stronger flavor. Fresh herbs are usually used in a cold infusion, especially smaller flowers and other delicate parts of the plant. However, be careful to dry the herbs thoroughly before using them, as water will encourage the growth of bacteria and mold in the oil. It is best to leave the herbs in the air for 24 hours so that excess water can evaporate off. This extraction is encouraged by sunlight, and it is best done with olive oil, as it is the least likely to turn rancid.

However, it is worth mentioning that many herbs like lemon balm and St John's wort lose much of their benefits when dried. use fresh, although wilted, herbs all the time.

A well-made oil has little or no water in it to grow mold. The problem is people are putting fresh herbs in oil and then sealing the jar. You should use dried herbs if you're going to do that. The right procedure with fresh herbs is to cover the top of jar with a coffee filter or cheese cloth then heat it or leave under the sun for up to 48 hours. It doesn't matter whether you choose to use the sun or artificial heat. I like my crockpot on the lowest to evaporate the water and infuse the oil. When you have taken this extra step with fresh herbs, strain, cap tightly and store in dark place.

Here is what you need:
10.

- A Clean and Clear Glass Jar with a Lid

- A Wide-Mouthed Jug

- A Muslin Bag

- A Dark Glass Bottle

- A Funnel

- Herbs

- Oil

To infuse herbal oil the cold way, follow these steps:

1. Place dried herbs in a sterilized jar. For a decent batch, add about 500 g (17.6 oz) of herbs.

2. Pour about 2 cups of olive oil over the herbs.

3. Close the jar, securing tightly, and give it a few good shakes.

4. Place the jar someplace sunny, like a windowsill, and let it sit for two to six weeks. Shake occasionally.

5. Place the muslin bag over the jug, securing it over the rim

and tucking the middle of the cloth inside.

6. Pour the oil through the muslin, and bring the edges of the cloth together, trapping the herbs inside. Keep squeezing until all the liquid is strained.

7. With the help of a funnel, pour the strained oil into a dark glass bottle. Use as needed.

Dosage: Unless the herbs used come with special precautions or concerns about your unique condition, you should be free to apply or consume the oil as much as you think is necessary.

Storage: Store the bottles somewhere dry and dark for up to one year. For best results, make a habit of using the oil within six months, as after that the oil will start losing its medicinal powers.

Note: So, keep in mind that most herbs work well dried but a few need to be used fresh. That is one reason you need to know your plant. Some Herbs need to be fresh when the oil is added, because, their oils need to be infused in the carrier oil instead of evaporating. For instance, dried lemon had some value for relieving depression but not much value against Herpes virus unless fresh. Much of its medicinal value is in the plant's oils. If you make the infused oil with fresh herb, it has multiple uses instead of limited uses.

If you are unsure about your herbs or the procedures, you are very welcome to join our private herbal community in Facebook and get advice from other herbalists. You will find the QR code at the end of this book. You scan the QR code with your camera and it takes you to our group. You can also just search "Herbalism For Beginners At Home – Medicinal Herbs and Herbalist Remedies" and request to join our group.

Essential Oils

In the past, essential oils were where I drew the line. I could whip up creams, tinctures and infusions, but making essential oils was something I always steered away from. That is until I developed the confidence to give it a try! Homemade essential oils are not only cost effective, especially if you have an herb garden, but they can also be very rewarding to make. There is something empowering about being able to say, "Here, try the essential oil I've made."

As challenging as the process may sound, it is actually very simple. If you think about it, essential oils are no more than products distilled from steam. You just simmer the herb, the steam goes through a tube, the tube runs through cold water, condensation occurs, and that's it. Your essential oil is born.

And you don't need tons of fancy ingredients either. You can do it with just a few essentials:

- A Crockpot with a Lid
- Distilled Water
- 3–4 cups of Fresh Herbs
- Small Dark Glass Bottles
- A Turkey Baster
- A Stove

Ready to give it a try? Here are the steps to making your first essential oil:

1. Chop up your preferred herbs, using enough to fill the crockpot about ¾ of the way. Usually, about 3–4 cups of plant material should suffice.

2. Pour enough distilled water into the crockpot to cover the chopped herbs.

3. Place the lid on but put it <u>upside down</u>. This is important, as the lid's concave curves will push the steam back inside. Alternatively, you can use a plate for this purpose.

4. Place the crockpot over high heat and cook until the water becomes very hot. Then turn the heat to low and allow the herbs to simmer for a good three to four hours.

5. Remove from heat and allow to cool completely.

6. Transfer to the fridge and leave it there overnight.

7. The next day, when uncovering the pot, you will notice that a thin, oily film has formed on top of the liquid. That's

your essential oil. This layer will be slightly hardened and you need to gather it quickly as it will soon start to melt away, as the pot warms up to room temperature. For extra precision, use a turkey baster for this step. It will be like lifting excess fat from the top of the gravy. Then fill up your sterilized dark glass bottles.

8. If you don't follow these steps correctly, you might notice some water-based liquid at the bottom of the bottle of essential oil. If this bothers you, you can reheat the oil so that the water will become steam and escape from the bottle. If you do that, be super gentle; essential oils lose their potency when heated, so don't overdo it.

Always use fresh herbs for this extraction method, as the dried versions will contain significantly less essential oil. Chopping the plants is also crucial, to increase the surface area from which oils can escape the herbs.

Storage: Secured tightly, the glass bottles should be stored in a dark and cool place. You can generally use them for up to a year, but after the first six months the essential oils will begin to lose their potency.

Tonic Wines

Tonic wines are the best way to extract the medicinal properties from tonic herbs, and the most effective method for supporting digestion and improving vitality. Angelica, especially Chinese dong quai angelica, is one of the most popular herbal ingredients for making a red or white wine tonic.

The key to making an especially potent tonic wine is to keep oxygen exposure to a minimum. That is why I don't recommend doing this in bottles, jugs, or pots that will be opened and exposed to the atmosphere regularly. Herbs soaked in wine will turn moldy if they are frequently in contact with air. To prevent this from happening, I suggest using a jar with a tap at the base. That way, you have control over the flow of wine without exposing the mixture to the air or upsetting the herbs.

To make a tonic wine, you will need:

- 1 liter (1 quart) of Red or White Wine

- 100 g (3.5 oz) of Dried Tonic Herbs or 25–30 g (1 oz) of Dried Bitter Herbs

- A Clean Jar with a Tap at the Base

Steps to making a tonic wine:

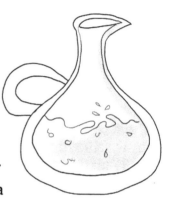

1. Place the dried herbs inside a sterilized jar.

2. Pour the wine over the herbs, keeping in mind that the wine should cover the herbs completely.

3. Close the jar tightly and give it a gentle shake.

4. Let the jar sit for two to six weeks so that the herbs can soak and the wine can become more mature.

Dosage: After the maturation period is over and two to six weeks have passed, tap off about ⅓ cup, and drink before a meal. I do this once a day before dinner, but you can do so before lunch as well, especially if you have digestive issues.

Storage: If stored properly, the wine will be safe to consume for at least three months. If the wine takes on a funny flavor and aroma, it may signify that the herbs have become moldy or the wine has oxidized. If that happens, discard the remedy, and steep yourself a new batch.

Poultices

When I'm making poultices, I always feel like a Victorian nurse using my herbalist powers to relieve someone's condition. Once you try your hand at whipping up these soothing mixtures, you will also begin to feel like a herbal healer. As simple as this method is, it can be ten times more effective than other methods we have discussed.

Poultices are a simple mix of fresh, powdered, or dried herbs, simmered and applied to an affected area on the skin. The herbs' active substances will seep through the skin and do their magic to ease nerve or muscle pain and promote healing.

To make your own poultice, you will need:

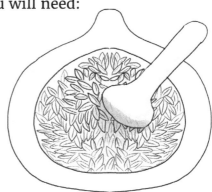

- A Saucepan

- Some Gauze

- A Little Bit of Water

- A Few Drops of Oil

- A Stove

And here is how you can do it:

1. Place your herbs in the saucepan and add a bit of water to the pan. Don't go overboard, but use a sufficient amount. There should be enough water to cover the affected area of your skin.

2. Place saucepan over medium heat and simmer for two to three minutes.

3. Scoop the herbs up with a spoon and carefully squeeze the excess liquid from them. You can do this with a second spoon or by pressing the mixture in your hands.

4. Rub a few drops of oil onto the affected area to prevent the herbs from sticking to the skin.

5. Apply the simmered herbs, while still hot, onto the location, and place the gauze over the top of the herbs, tying it securely to make sure the herbs stay in contact.

6. Leave for two to three hours, or as needed.

Application: Every two or three hours, apply a new poultice until the condition's severity subsides.

Ointments

The thing that makes ointments so effective is that they use fatty ingredients and absolutely no water. These applications can form a protective layer over the skin, which is especially useful when treating inflammation or damaged surfaces. The point is for the ointment to keep moisture at bay, sealing the skin off from water and the environment. This is why ointments are so helpful with treating conditions like diaper rash.

I used to think it was impossible to replace store-bought ointments with homemade herbal remedies, but this recipe for ointment will convince any skeptic otherwise.

Here is what you need:

- A Double Boiler (Or a Saucepan and a Heat-Resistant Bowl)
- Herb-infused Oil of Choice
- Beeswax
- A Wooden Spatula
- Small Dark Glass Jars with Lids

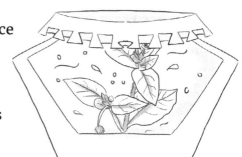

Method of preparation for ointments:

1. Melt wax in double boiler, or in the heat-resistant bowl placed over a saucepan containing warm water.

2. Add oil. Use 1 cup herb-infused oil to 2 tablespoons beeswax.

3. Remove from the heat and stir till cool enough to stay emulsified (combined).

4. Pour into containers and cool completely.

Beeswax can be difficult to clean out of your double boiler and so, to avoid this tiresome problem, I use a small can that I place in a saucepan containing a little warm water. This works in a similar manner to a water bath. The advantage is that, once I have finished working with the beeswax, I leave the remainder in the can to harden. I cover the can and leave it until the next time I wish to make an ointment. This saves contaminating your double boiler with sticky beeswax.

A salve is a thicker version of an ointment. It is made in the same way as described above, but the ratio of beeswax to oil should be 1:2. If you wish, you can use part coconut oil when you make the original herb-infused oil for your ointment or salve. Ointments and salves should stay on top of the skin to protect damaged areas, and the active ingredients should be absorbed into the body for the soothing, pain-relieving properties to have their effect.

Dosage: Apply a small amount of the ointment onto the affected area, three times a day. If you are using an ointment to treat diaper rash, apply it with every diaper change.

Storage: Store your tightly closed dark glass jars in a cool and dark spot, and use within three months.

Creams

Unlike ointments that are water-free, creams are mixtures of fat and water. They do not offer a protective layer on the surface but blend with the skin. The medicinal properties provide a cooling or soothing effect. In this way, the skin is allowed to breathe and can heal much more quickly.

I've found that my creams are most beneficial and much gentler when made with a wax and glycerin combination. You could use a traditional glycerite, which is a fluid extract of an herb, made using glycerin as part of the extraction medium. I am sharing my secret recipe with you now.

You will need:

- A Saucepan and Heat-Resistant Glass Bowl, or a Small Double Boiler

- A Wooden Spatula

- A Muslin Bag
- A Jug or Pot
- A Spread Knife
- Small Dark Glass Jars
- Beeswax
- Glycerin and Herbs (or Glycerite of Choice)
- Water

The method:

1. Fill a saucepan half way with water and place over high heat. Bring to a boil.

2. Lower the heat to a simmer and rest a glass bowl over the pan. Or use a double boiler instead.

3. Add about 150 g (5.3 oz) of beeswax to the bowl and stir until melted.

4. Then, stir in the glycerin; about 75 g (2.7 oz), or ½ the amount of wax.

5. Add ⅓ cup of water to the mix.

6. Stir in about 30 g (1.05 oz) of dried herbs and cover the glass bowl.

7. Leave the mixture to heat gently, over the hot water of the saucepan, for three full hours.

8. Secure the muslin bag over a jug or pot and pour the herb mixture through to strain it.

9. Bring the edges of the bag together and squeeze to push the strained liquid into the jug.

10. Stir gently as the mixture cools and the cream sets.

11. Have your sterilized dark glass jars ready and transfer the cream into the jars with the help of a small spread knife.

12. Secure tightly and store in refrigerator until needed.

Tip: You can also add extra ingredients to your creams such as powders, tinctures, or essential oils for an added medicinal boost.

Dosage: Apply the cream to the affected area up to three times a day.

Storage: Unlike ointments, creams deteriorate quickly due to the water content. They should be stored in the fridge. If secured tightly, they should last for a good three months.

Compresses

After my usual hiking misadventures and clumsiness, I often come home with a swollen ankle or a particularly bruised knee. After returning, I take a relaxing shower, put my leg up, apply a compress onto the affected area, and enjoy a cup of herbal infusion or tea.

A compress is just a cloth that has been soaked in an herbal infusion or decoction, and then applied onto an injury or bruise to promote healing or alleviate pain.

To make a compress, you will need:

– A Clean Bowl

– Clean Soft Cloth or Washcloth

– Infusion, Decoction or Tincture and Water Mix

Method for preparing a compress:

1. Prepare your infusion or decoction, strain well, and let it cool so it is not unbearably hot. For a compress, you will need about 2 cups of infusion or decoction. You can also make this with a tincture. If you are using a tincture, combine 5 tsp of tincture in 2 cups of water.

2. Pour the infusion, decoction or diluted tincture into a clean bowl.

3. Soak the clean cloth completely in the infused liquid, then

wring out the excess.

4. Place the soaked cloth onto the affected area. You can even secure it with some safety pins or string.

5. Re-soak as it cools and replace. The warmth will feel good and improve the absorption of the herb(s).

6. Leave for one to two hours.

Instead of applying the compress, you can also use a lotion bath for the same purpose. Instead of placing the cloth over the area after wringing out the excess liquid, just wring out the liquid directly over the affected area. Soak, wring, bathe, repeat. Soon, you will have the desired results.

Application: Use as needed.

Storage: Store the compress infusions in clean bottles in the fridge for up to 48 hours.

Powders, Capsules, Pills

Powdered herbs are just that – herbs that have been ground to a powdered consistency. Usually, a mortar and pestle are used for making powders, but anything that can finely grind can be used for this purpose. Although powders can be sprinkled over food as spices, or even taken with water, one of the most convenient ways to consume an herbal supplement is in capsule form, or rolled into pills.

However, not all herbs can be finely powdered at home. Some may require a more forceful approach; for such herbs, I suggest buying the powdered versions. Most herbal suppliers should be well-stocked with powdered herbs. For making capsules, I recommend looking for a very fine grade of powdered herbs. You will also need empty capsules, which are sold in both gelatin and vegetarian form, in most specialist outlets.

To make capsules you will need:

– A Saucer

- Powdered Herbs

- Empty Capsules

And this is how you can make capsules:

1. Pour the powdered herb into a saucer.

2. Holding two empty capsule halves, scoop the powder up by sliding the capsule halves towards each other.

3. Once you have filled the capsule cases, gently slide them together, keeping the powder locked inside.

For a 00-size capsule, you will need about 250 mg of powder. If this is something you decide to do often, you could consider purchasing a small machine that will help you fill many capsules in a short time; also, it packs the powdered herb so tightly that a 00-size capsule holds up to 450 mg.

Dosage: Depending on the herb used, take two to three capsules a day.

Storage: Place the capsules in dark glass containers and store them in a dark and cool place for up to three or four months.

To make pills you will need:

- A Small Bowl
- Powdered Herbs
- Binding Agent such as Honey or Gum Tragacanth
- Oven

And this is how you can make your own pills:

1. Pour your powdered herbs into the small bowl.

2. Add a teaspoon of honey (or other binding agent) and enough water to make a paste that resembles bread dough.

3. Roll out into the shape of a long, thin rope.

4. Cut the rope into small segments. (You can now roll each segment in a powdered spice of your choice, such as

cinnamon.)

5. Place the pills onto a baking tray and dry them in a cool oven.

Dosage: Depending on the herb used, take two to three pills a day.

Storage: The pills should be stored in a dry and cool place in a dark glass jar up to four months.

Steam Inhalations

Steam inhalations are my go-to remedy for the sinus-related troubles caused by seasonal allergies. These inhalations are an effective way to clear congestion, especially when using herbs that have antiseptic medical actions, such as goldenseal, thyme, or myrrh.

To make a steam inhalation, you will need:

- 25–30 g (1 oz) of Preferred Herbs
- 1 Liter of Water (1 Quart)
- A Pot
- A Towel
- A Stove

And the method for creating a steam inhalation is quite simple:

1. Heat the water to a boil before pouring over the herb leaves or flowers.

2. Allow to steep for 15 minutes.

3. If you are using roots or barks, which release their goodies when simmered, you should simmer for 15 minutes, then allow cool for a further 15 minutes.

4. Reheat liquid to simmer (a bit cooler than a boil).

5. Remove the pot from the heat.

6. Place your head over the pot, and cover both your head and the bowl with the towel.

7. Close your eyes, and stay in this position, inhaling steam for approximately ten minutes.

Remember that high heat destroys the value in many herbs; I recommend to never boil herbs, but to just simmer them. I strongly advise you not to rush the process of using a steam inhalation. If you're impatient like me, you can put on some music to help you relax. I also recommend not leaving the room for about 15 minutes, even after the inhalation process is complete. This is so that you can further support the clearing of congestion.

Mouth Gargles and Washes

Mouthwashes and gargles are usually used to treat infections and inflammation of the mouth and throat. They are most effective with herbs that have astringent compounds, such as myrrh, as they can heal and repair the mucous membrane. To make them more beneficial for the throat, you can also add a small amount of licorice to the mix.

To make a mouthwash or gargle, you will need:

- ⅓ Cup of Infusion

- A Glass

And here is how you do it:

1. Make an infusion with your preferred herbs, but do not strain right away. To increase the astringency, let the herbs sit in the saucepan for about 15 minutes longer.

2. Strain, as you normally would, and pour into a glass, only filling the glass about ⅓ of the way.

3. Gargle or rinse the mouth with small portions of the liquid.

The best thing about these homemade herbal gargles and mouthwashes is that they are made with natural and safe

ingredients through infusion or decoction. This means that you don't need to worry about accidentally swallowing the liquid. On the contrary, doing so can further benefit your health.

Tip: You can also make a mouthwash by mixing ⅓ cup of hot water and 1 tsp (about 5 ml) of your preferred tincture.

Each of the above preparation methods allows healing substances in the herbs to be extracted differently and also results in different ways of applying the extract. While you can use an infusion for drinking, gargling, or placing onto an affected area as a compress, there is only one way of applying an ointment.

Before using any of these methods to address a health concern, make sure to inform yourself of the possible risks and side effects. While a syrup may present some benefit, that may not be the best application for your mouth sores. Similarly, a tincture of myrrh may not be helpful for your insomnia.

The next chapters will teach you all about pairing particular conditions with the right remedies, thereby removing all the guesswork involved in becoming a master of herbal healing.

Ailments and Their Herbal Remedies

erbal remedies can be a safer, more natural, and even a healthier alternative to conventional medication. Their effects depend on the condition's intensity and other factors that are unique to each individual; generally, herbs provide a powerful and efficient healing base. Some ailments may need a chemical approach, of course, but for most health issues, the cure lies in nature. Here are the most common 71 health concerns that can be treated easily with natural, plant-based remedies. For each ailment, I have suggested only a small sample of the many different herbs that can be used for treatment. There are many other remedies out there and each human body reacts best to a certain remedy. You will get to know what works best for your body by experimenting with different herbs, one at a time.

#1 Anemia
Herb: Nettle

Remedy: Make nettle infusion and drink 3 cups a day.

#2 Anxiety
Herb: Valerian, Hops

Remedies: Add about 10 drops of valerian tincture into water and drink, a couple of times a day, for two weeks. For excessive anxiety, make a hops tincture and dilute 20 drops of the tincture into a glass of water. Take this mixture up to six times a day.

#3 Acne
Herbs:

Calendula, Comfrey, Echinacea
Remedies: Calendula and comfrey cream can be applied to the affected area twice a day. In addition, you can consume one echinacea tablet a day for several weeks.

#4 Allergies
Herbs: Nettle, Elderflower
Remedies: Take 1–2 cups of a nettle infusion each day for three months; or use 1 cup elderflower infusion each day, starting one month before the hay fever season, and continuing for its duration.

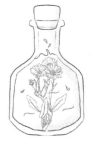

#5 Asthma
Herb: Echinacea, Nettle, Thyme
Remedies: For shortness of breath, concoct a nettle and thyme infusion, and take about 3 cups a day; for mild bronchial asthma, make echinacea tablets and take one daily.

#6 Athlete's Foot
Herbs: Turmeric, Calendula
Remedy: Make a calendula ointment and combine 3 tsp of the ointment with ½ tsp of turmeric powder. Rub the affected area daily.

#7 Backache
Herbs: St. John's Wort, Lavender, Rosemary, Thyme
Remedies: Make 3 cups of a thyme infusion, add to the warm water in a bath, and soak for 20 minutes; combine 20 drops of lavender essential oil, 2 tbsp St. John's Wort infused oil, and 10 drops of rosemary essential oil, and rub into the tense area.

#8 Bee Sting
Herbs: Lavender, Nettle
Remedy: Rub nettle leaf on the sting area (after removing the stinger) or apply lavender essential oil or tincture, for relief.

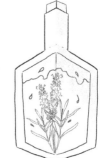

#9 Bloating
Herbs: Fennel, Peppermint
Remedies: Make a fennel infusion by combining ½ tsp of fennel seeds and ¾ cup of water. Drink this infusion three times a day; or consume 1 cup of a peppermint infusion one to three

times a day.

#10 Bronchitis
Herb: Echinacea
Remedy: Combine ½ tsp of echinacea tincture with some water, and drink two to three times a day. Alternatively, you can take one echinacea tablet daily.

#11 Bruises
Herbs: Arnica
Remedy: Apply an arnica ointment onto the affected area two to three times a day, but only if the skin is not broken.

#12 Burns
Herbs: Aloe Vera, Lavender, Calendula
Remedies: Apply aloe vera gel or lavender essential oil onto the affected area after the heat is gone. Repeat as needed. Make a calendula infusion and apply it cold onto the affected area.

#13 Chapped Lips
Herb: Elderflower
Remedy: Make a cream or ointment from elderflowers and apply the mixture onto chapped lips. It should work well on any chapped surface of your skin.

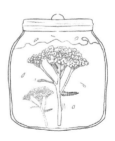

#14 Canker Sore
Herb: Myrrh
Remedy: Combine ½ tsp of myrrh tincture with 3 tsp of water and gargle for one minute.

#15 Chickenpox
Herbs: Echinacea, St. John's Wort, Lemon Balm
Remedy: Take about half a teaspoon of echinacea tincture with some water, and drink it a couple of times a day. This will boost the immune system. In addition, take half a teaspoon of lemon balm tincture, or make a salve with lemon balm oil. Lemon balm is particularly successful against the virus that causes chickenpox. Lastly, half a teaspoon of St. John's wort tincture in water, or a cream made with St. John's wort tincture, will help soothe itching and pain.

#16 Cold

<u>Herb</u>: Ginger

<u>Remedy</u>: Infuse 3 slices of fresh ginger in ¾ cup of water. Drink three times a day.

#17 Cold Sore

<u>Herb</u>: Lemon Balm

<u>Remedies</u>: Make a lemon balm Infusion and sip throughout the day, consuming no more than 3 cups. You can also infuse 3 tsp of fresh or freshly dried lemon balm in ¾ cup water for ten minutes to use externally. Strain, let cool and then dab onto the affected area three times a day.

#18 Colic

<u>Herb</u>: Fennel

<u>Remedy</u>: Combine 1 level tsp of fennel seeds and ¾ cups of water. Simmer for ten minutes, strain, allow to cool slightly and offer to your baby. It is healthy to drink up to one cup per day.

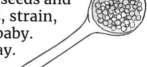

#19 Conjunctivitis

<u>Herb</u>: German Chamomile

<u>Remedy</u>: Infuse two German Chamomile tea bags in two cups of water. Allow to cool, squeeze out the excess tea, and place the teabags over the eyes.

#20 Constipation

<u>Herbs</u>: Peppermint, Ginger, Dandelion, Licorice

<u>Remedies</u>: Teas and infusions made from any combination of the herbs mentioned above can be powerful for battling constipation. Drink 2–3 cups a day.

#21 Cough

<u>Herb</u>: Thyme

<u>Remedy</u>: Make a thyme infusion and consume 3 cups a day.

#22 Dandruff

<u>Herb</u>: Tea Tree

<u>Remedy</u>: Dilute a few drops of tea tree essential oil in your regular shampoo, and wash your hair as usual. Do not apply tea tree oil undiluted directly on the scalp. This usage can cause inflammation and rashes.

#23 Diaper Rash

<u>Herbs</u>: Chickweed, Calendula
<u>Remedies</u>: Make chickweed ointment and apply once or twice a day. Calendula ointment can be applied to dry skin each time you're changing a diaper.

#24 Diarrhea

<u>Herb</u>: Agrimony
<u>Remedy</u>: Drink about 1 ½ cups of an agrimony infusion each day for three days.

#25 Digestive Inflammation Including GERD (Gastroesophageal Reflux Disease)

<u>Herb</u>: Licorice
<u>Remedy</u>: Make a licorice tincture and combine ½ tsp of this tincture with ½ cup of water. Drink twice a day.

#26 Earache

<u>Herb</u>: Lavender, Garlic, Mullein
<u>Remedy</u>: Place a couple of drops of lavender essential oil onto a cotton ball and place it inside the affected ear as a plug. Keep the cotton ball in place for at least 10–15 minutes. Garlic-Mullein ear oil is an even more effective remedy, used in the same way. Do not drop undiluted essential oils directly into the ear canal.

#27 Eczema

<u>Herb</u>: German Chamomile, Witch Hazel

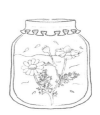

<u>Remedies</u>: Make about 3 cups of chamomile infusion. Add this infusion to a bath while it is still hot, and soak for 15–25 minutes. You can also allow the infusion to cool and apply it to the itchy area as a compress. You can also use a witch hazel cream, applying it to the affected area up to five times a day.

#28 Fatigue

<u>Herbs</u>: Ginseng, St. John's Wort
<u>Remedies</u>: Make ginseng capsules and take up to 1 g of powder a day. Make a St. John's wort infusion and consume no more than 2⅓ cups a day.

#29 Fever
Herbs: Yarrow, Elderberry
Remedy: Infuse ½ tsp each of yarrow and elderberry in ⅓ cup of water. Brew for ten minutes and drink five to six times a day. Do not consume more than 2⅓ cups a day.

#30 Flu
Herbs: Thyme, Elderflower, Lemon Balm
Remedy: Place about 1½–2 tbsp of each herb in 3 cups of water. Brew for ten minutes and drink up. Do not consume more than 3 cups a day.

#31 Fractures
Herb: Comfrey
Remedies: Make comfrey ointment or cream, and apply these mixtures to the affected area, three to four times a day, as long as the skin is not broken. Alternatively, you can make a comfrey infusion and apply cold compresses to the area.

#32 Gastritis
Herb: Goldenseal
Remedies: Make goldenseal capsules with goldenseal powder and take one, three times a day. Alternatively, you can drink 2 cups of goldenseal infusion daily. Note that this can be VERY bitter.

#33 Gingivitis (Gum Inflammation)
Herb: Myrrh
Remedy: Using the same remedy as was used for canker sores, combine ½ tsp of myrrh tincture and 3 tsp of water, and gargle for a minute.

#34 Hair Loss
Herb: Thyme
Remedy: Make a thyme infusion, allow to cool, and massage the warm mixture into the scalp to reverse hair loss and support hair growth.

#35 Halitosis (Bad Breath)
Herb: Tea Tree, Sage
Remedy: Dilute one drop of tea tree oil in a couple of vegetable oil drops and add it to a cup of warm water. Rinse your mouth with some of the solution for 30 seconds and spit out. Do this until you have used the entire cup. Alternatively, make 1 cup of sage Infusion, rinse your mouth with some of the solution for 30

seconds and spit out. Rinse and repeat until the cup is empty.

#36 Hangover
Herb: Dandelion
Remedy: Make a decoction with 15 g (½ oz) of dandelion root and 3 cups of water. Drink, in small quantities, frequently during the day.

#37 Headache
Herbs: Rosemary, Lavender
Remedies: Make a rosemary infusion and drink 2 cups a day. As a general headache remedy, you can also rub lavender or rosemary essential oil on the temples for a couple of minutes to relax and calm the pain in your head.

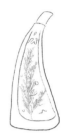

#38 Hemorrhoids
Herb: Witch Hazel
Remedy: Apply witch hazel ointment after each bowel movement, or once to twice a day.

#39 High Blood Pressure
Herbs: Garlic, Ginkgo
Remedies: Eat one to two fresh garlic cloves each day, or take one garlic tablet daily. As an alternative, take one ginkgo tablet a day for two to three months

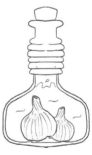

#40 Hives
Herbs: Chickweed, Nettle
Remedies: Apply chickweed cream to the affected area or make a nettle infusion and drink it regularly throughout the day, consuming no more than 3 cups in total.

#41 Indigestion
Herb: German Chamomile, Fennel
Remedy: Make a chamomile, or a fennel seed infusion and drink 1 cup after each meal, or as needed.

#42 Insect Bites
Herbs: Sage, Basil, Thyme
Remedy: Extract the juice from the leaves of one of the herbs

above and apply directly onto the bites.

#43 Insomnia
<u>Herbs</u>: Lavender, Chamomile, Valerian
<u>Remedies</u>: Make a lavender infusion and drink ¾ cup before bedtime. Alternatively, take 1 cup of chamomile infusion before going to bed. For a more intense state of insomnia, make valerian tablets, and take one before going to bed.

#44 Liver Infections
<u>Herb</u>: Milk Thistle
<u>Remedy</u>: Make a milk thistle decoction and drink about ⅓ cup a day.

#45 Menopause
<u>Herbs</u>: Sage, Black Cohosh
<u>Remedies</u>: Make a sage infusion
and drink one cup at night to reduce night sweats and hot flashes. In addition, you can also take one black cohosh tablet to tackle fluctuating estrogen and progesterone levels.

#46 Mental Focus
<u>Herb</u>: Ginkgo
<u>Remedy</u>: Make ginkgo tablets and take one daily.

#47 Muscle Cramps
<u>Herb</u>: Arnica
<u>Remedy</u>: Make an arnica cream or ointment, and apply it to the affected area, massaging for a minute or two.

#48 Nausea
<u>Herb</u>: Lemon Balm
<u>Remedy</u>: Make a lemon balm infusion using dried herbs and drink 2–3 cups a day.

#49 Period Pain
<u>Herb</u>: Black Cohosh
<u>Remedy</u>: Make a black cohosh tincture and combine 40 drops of this mixture with ½ cup of water. Drink three times a day.

#50 Premenstrual Syndrome (PMS)
<u>Herbs</u>: Vervain, Rosemary
<u>Remedies</u>: Make vervain tablets and take one daily. Add 5–10

drops of rosemary essential oil to a bath and soak for twenty minutes.

#51 Psoriasis
Herb: Turmeric
Remedy: Make a poultice with 1 tsp of turmeric powder and a just enough water to form a paste. Apply directly to the affected area, three times a day. Be careful as turmeric stains, especially clothes.

#52 Rheumatoid Arthritis
Herb: Black Cohosh
Remedy: Make a black cohosh decoction, and sip throughout the day, consuming up to 3 cups each day.

#53 Shingles
Herbs: Garlic, Ginger, Lemon Balm
Remedies: Apply fresh ginger or garlic slices onto unopened shingles up to six times a day. Make a lemon balm infusion and drink 2–3 cups daily. Alternatively, a salve made with lemon balm can be applied to the shingles and this will help fight the virus that causes the condition.

#54 Sinus Infection
Herb: German Chamomile, Thyme
Remedy: Make a steam inhalation with 15 g (½ ounce) of chamomile or thyme in 3 cups of water. Place your head over the pot with the infusion, throw a towel over both your head and the pot, and inhale for ten minutes.

#55 Skin Tags
Herb: Tea Tree
Remedy: Add a few drops of tea tree essential oil to a cotton ball and apply it onto the skin tag, letting it rest there for about ten minutes. A piece of sticking plaster will help to keep it in place. Do this three times a day for as long as it takes for the tag to fall off.

#56 Sore Muscles
Herbs: Thyme, Rosemary

Remedy: Make 3 cups of infusion with one (or both) of the herbs and add the hot water to a bath. Soak for about 20 minutes

#57 Sore Throat
Herbs: Rosemary, Myrrh, Echinacea
Remedy: Add ⅓ tsp of each herb to 5 tsp of warm water, mix to combine, and gargle for a minute. Do not swallow if pregnant.

#58 Sprains
Herb: Arnica, Comfrey
Remedy: Make arnica cream or ointment, apply to the affected area, and massage in for a few minutes. Do this three times a day. Make a comfrey poultice and apply to the sprain.

#59 Stiff Joints
Herbs: St. John's Wort, Lavender
Remedy: Combine about 2 ½ tbsp of St. John's wort-infused oil with 20–30 drops of lavender essential oil and massage the mixture into the stiff area.

#60 Stomach Spasms
Herbs: German Chamomile, Angelica
Remedy: Make an infusion with three parts of chamomile and one part of angelica root. Sip throughout the day, consuming up to 3 cups.

#61 Stress
Herb: Ginseng
Remedy: Take one to two ginseng capsules a day.

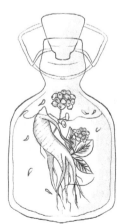

#62 Sunburn
Herb: Aloe Vera
Remedy: Apply aloe vera gel to the sunburned area as often as necessary.

#63 Swelling and Fluid Retention
Herb: Dandelion
Remedies: Make dandelion leaf infusion and drink 2 cups a day. You can also make dandelion juice from the leaves of the plant, and consume 1 tbsp of the juice three times a day.

#64 Tongue Ulcers

<u>Herbs</u>: Myrrh, Licorice, Echinacea

<u>Remedies</u>: Combine equal parts of the tinctures of the herbs and apply neatly onto the area of the mouth. Alternatively, dilute one part of the tincture mixture in five parts water and gargle.

#65 Tonsillitis

<u>Herb</u>: Echinacea

<u>Remedy</u>: Make echinacea tablets and take one to two each day. Take no more than 1 g of powder a day.

#66 Travel Sickness

<u>Herbs</u>: Ginger, Turmeric

<u>Remedy</u>: Make an infusion with 2 slices of ginger and ½ tsp of turmeric powder in ¾ cup of water. Drink no more than 3 cups a day. Alternatively, eat candied ginger, or the powdered ginger spice in your kitchen!

#67 Urinary Tract Infection (UTI)

<u>Herbs</u>: Garlic, Echinacea

<u>Remedy</u>: Make tablets or capsules of either or both herbs and take one each day.

#68 Varicose Veins

<u>Herbs</u>: Calendula, Witch Hazel

<u>Remedy</u>: Combine equal parts of calendula and witch hazel cream and apply to the affected area.

#69 Warts

<u>Herb</u>: Aloe Vera, Tea Tree

<u>Remedy</u>: Apply aloe vera gel onto the wart a couple of times a day for up to three months. You can also dilute 1–2 drops of tea tree essential oil in 12 drops of almond oil, and apply 3–4 drops of the mixture to a cotton ball that you place on the wart. Repeat two or three times a day.

#70 Wounds

<u>Herbs</u>: Comfrey, Aloe Vera

<u>Remedy</u>: Make comfrey ointment and apply around the edges of the wounded area. Once you see that a scab has formed, cleanse with aloe vera gel.

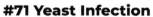

#71 Yeast Infection

<u>Herb</u>: Calendula

<u>Remedy</u>: Make 3 cups of calendula infusion and add, while still warm, to a bath. Soak for 15–25 minutes.

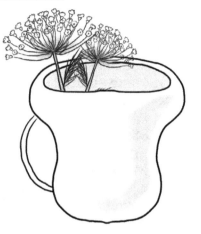

Handy Herbal Recipes and Mixtures

lthough we have already covered 15 extraction methods that can be used to prepare all types of herbal cures, and been through a whopping 71 remedies that will help with the process of healing, it would be remiss not to treat you to some herbal recipes. Think of this chapter as your final lesson in becoming a master herbal healer, in which you finish off your training and invoke your strengths. This final chapter should inspire you to be bold and make your own colorful herbal creations.

Rosemary and Ginger Tea With Lemon to Strengthen Your Immune System

Ingredients:
1 Slice of Lemon
1 tbsp Sliced Fresh Ginger
1 tsp Chopped Rosemary
1 cup Water

Method:
1. Combine the ginger and water in a small pot, and place over medium heat.

2. Simmer for about five minutes to decoct, then turn off the heat.

3. Add the rosemary and cover the pot. Allow to infuse for ten minutes.

4. Strain the mixture and squeeze the lemon juice into the pot just before serving. Enjoy!

Tea for Reduced Heart Rate and Lower Blood Pressure

Ingredients:
1 ⅓ tbsp Dried Nettle Leaves
1 ⅓ tbsp Dried Elderberry
1 ⅓ tbsp Dried Lemon Balm
1 ⅓ tbsp Dried Hawthorne Berries
1 liter (1 quart) of Water

Method:
1. Bring the water to a boil and remove the pot from heat.

2. Add the herbs to the pot, and cover.

3. Let sit for five minutes, then strain into a clean bottle.

4. Drink about 3 tbsp of the tea approximately every hour or so for 12 days straight.

Weight-Loss Tea

Ingredients:
1 tbsp Dried Nettle Leaves
½ tbsp Dried Orange Peel
½ tbsp Sliced Ginger
½ tbsp Dried Dandelion Leaves
¼ tbsp Fennel Seeds
2 ½ cups Water

Method:
1. Bring 2 ½ cups of water to a boil, then remove from heat.

2. Add the herbs, cover the pot, and let sit for three to five minutes.

3. Strain into a bottle and consume during the day.

Mental Relief Tincture

Ingredients:
1 liter (1 quart) Vodka
5 tbsp Dried Valerian Root
2 tbsp Chopped Rosemary
1 tbsp Chopped Peppermint

Method:
1. Place all the ingredients in a sterilized jar.

2. Seal the jar well and shake to combine.

3. Place in a dark and cool spot and allow to sit for three weeks. Make sure to shake the jar well once a day.

4. Start with ¼ of a tablespoon mixed with some water, and then take additional doses after 30 minutes if needed.

Ginger and Elderberry Tonic for Winter Vitality

Ingredients:
2 cups Water
1 cup Dried Elderberries
1 tbsp Grated Fresh Ginger
½ cup Raw Honey
1 tsp of Your Favorite Spice (Cinnamon works well for me)

Method:
1. Place the ginger, elderberries, and water in a pot.

2. Place over medium heat and bring just barely to a boil.

3. Reduce the heat to low, then allow the mixture to simmer for 20 minutes or so.

4. Allow to cool until safe to handle and strain the liquid through a sieve.

5. Stir in the honey and spice and pour into a clean glass jar or bottle.

6. Store in the fridge and enjoy 1 tablespoon a day.

Mouth Wash Mixture (Perfect for Inflammation)

Ingredients:
1 tbsp Dried St. John's Wort
1 tbsp Dried Nettle
1 tbsp Dried Chamomile
¾ liter (¾ quart) Boiling Water

Method:

1. Place the herbs in a small pot and pour the boiling water over them.

2. Cover and let sit for five minutes.

3. Strain the mixture into a clean glass jar or bottle with a lid

4. Gargle before and after each meal.

Herb-Infused Massage Oil

Ingredients:
⅓ cup Fresh Calendula
⅓ cup Fresh St. John's Wort
⅓ cup Fresh Lavender
300 ml (about 10–11 oz) of a Carrier Oil such as Almond, Sesame or Coconut Oil.

Method:
1. Place the plant material inside a previously sterilized glass jar.

2. Pour the carrier oil over the herbs, making sure to leave about two fingers of space for the fresh herbs to expand. The herbs should be totally submerged; otherwise, mold may form.

3. Seal the jar and let it sit in a warm space (near a window is perfect) for 30–40 days.

4. Strain the oil through a cheesecloth and into a clean bottle.

5. Store the massage oil in a dark and cool place, and use it as needed.

Calendula and Lavender Hand Salve

Ingredients:
1 tbsp Dried Calendula
1 tbsp Dried Lavender
50–60 ml (2 oz) Coconut Oil
80–90 ml (3 oz) Olive Oil
50–60 g (2 oz) Shea Butter
50–60 g (2 oz) Beeswax Pellets

Method:

1. Place the coconut oil and olive oil in a small pot over medium heat and heat until completely melted. Remove from the heat.

2. Add the calendula and lavender, give the mixture a gentle stir, and let the herbs sit for half an hour to infuse.

3. Strain the oil through cheesecloth or a fine-mesh sieve, into a glass jar.

4. Place the shea butter and beeswax in the pot you used earlier and melt the mixture over medium heat.

5. Add the mixture to the infused oil and stir gently to combine.

6. Seal the jar and let the salve solidify completely before using.

Stay Safe

Herbal medicine is indeed safe and natural, but that doesn't mean that it should be approached with no precautions. Not all herbs are harmless, and not all of us have the same health and nutritional requirements. The herbal remedy's effect depends on the active constituents in the herbs and how they interact with your metabolism and your unique medical condition.

Obviously, we cannot possibly cover every minor health issue and discuss every single chemical found in herbs. However, there are general guidelines that each aspiring herbalist must know to ensure safe and effective treatments.

Stick to What You Know. Experimenting with herbs you haven't used before is not only unwise, but it can also have a catastrophic effect. Even if you are not allergic to the plant or the herb is generally safe to consume, there may still be severe side effects. Herbs interact with each other and with commercial medications, and can worsen certain conditions. Research the herb well, and make sure that your physical and emotional state can benefit from its use. Also, when trying new treatments, try one herb at a time in case you react to it. If you use a combination, you won't be able to identify which herb disagrees with you.

Consume Only Appropriate Doses. Even the safest herbs that you have been consuming as tea, your whole life, can prove to have a negative effect if taken in large quantities. The remedies and preparations in this book suggest medicinal doses that shouldn't be exceeded. Before making your own recipe or self-prescribing a remedy, do some research to pinpoint the exact dosages that are appropriate.

When in Doubt, Avoid. The toxicity of certain herbs is not to be toyed with. If you are not sure whether you are overusing a concocted potion, or you have any uncertainties regarding the remedy, do not use it.

Avoid Long-Term Commitments. There are hundreds of herbs that are extremely safe to use, but only in the short term. Do some research and see just how long you can safely use a certain herb internally and externally. The safest herbs can be used until the symptoms go away, but if there are no improvements after two or three weeks, consult with a professional practitioner.

Important: Do not determine the dose yourself, and always follow professional advice.

Special Precautions for Children. Although many herbs can be safely offered to children, I strongly suggest not giving herbal remedies to babies under six months, unless your doctor advises otherwise. Be extremely cautious when giving remedies to children, and keep in mind that the dose must be adjusted, as well. See below:

6–12 months: one-tenth adult dose
1–6 years: one-third adult dose
7–12 years: half adult dose

The perfect ratio for the adult dose is explained in the extraction methods under "Harnessing the Essence of Herbs."

Special Precautions for Pregnancy. During the first trimester, avoid all herbal medicine unless your OB/GYN advises otherwise. Avoid alcohol-based tinctures when pregnant and use only herbs that are absolutely safe while in this condition.

Special Precautions for Older People. Older people, especially those over 70 years, have a much slower metabolism. For that reason, it is recommended that they take ¾ of the recommended adult doses.

Be Careful with Essential Oils. Never take essential oils internally unless your doctor gives you the green light. When applying topically, it is always best to dilute the oils with a carrier oil (vegetable or almond oil work well) before applying to the affected area.

Consider Your Condition. When searching for a remedy that will work for you, you need to take into consideration how you are feeling, how much you weigh, what you are allergic to, and what conditions you wish to treat. Also, keep in mind that herbal remedies are usually NOT a quick fix. Most treat the cause, not the symptoms. And then one must remember that herbs should not be used for more than three months without a break and a re-evaluation. If they're not doing the job, there may be an underlying reason. Consult with a professional to find out what changes should be made.

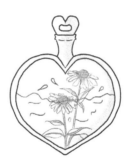

Conclusion

ongratulations! With the knowledge you've gathered under your belt, you are now officially eligible for trying your hand at some herbal healing.

After learning the basis of herbalism, getting acquainted with 40 of the essential herbs, discovering 15 different extraction methods, and becoming richer with the knowledge of many useful remedies and herbal recipes, it is safe to say that you now have what it takes to become an herbalist. So, feel free to go on a shopping spree for herbalism equipment, plant your herbal garden, and finally whip up plant-based medications for natural healing.

Now the time has come to reach for your mortar and pestle and grab some of your windowsill herbs! Find a simple remedy from this book and see how easy it is when you know what you are doing. From one herbalist to another, I salute your commitment and wish you a well-stocked home apothecary.

Just remember, you do not need much to embark on this journey into therapeutic healing, but you definitely need to travel safely if you want this healing journey to continue.

I'd love to hear all about your herbal adventures! Let's keep in touch! You will find your way to our herbal group below.

A Small Favor To Ask

My last request...

Being a smaller author, reviews help me tremendously! **It would mean the world to me** if you could leave a review!

If you liked reading this book and learned a thing or two, please scan the QR with your camera to leave a review!

Scan with your camera to leave a review!

Or email "greenhopexllc@gmail.com" with subject "Thank You Link" and I will send you the review link and our FB group link!

Have questions or need advice?
JOIN our <u>Herbal FAM JAM!</u>

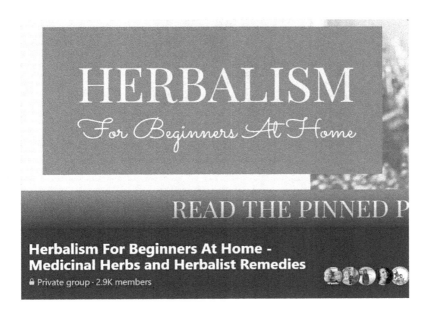

Connect with like-minded people in our private herbal community on Facebook.

Scan with your camera to join!

Or type this link

www.theherb.space/group

See the top herbalism books & other books by Ava

www.theherb.space/books

References and Further Reading

Agrawal, M., Nandini, D., Sharma, V., & Chauhan, N. S. (2010). Herbal remedies for treatment of hypertension. *International Journal of Pharmaceutical Sciences and Research 1* (5), pp. 1–21. http://dx.doi.org/10.13040/IJPSR.0975-8232.1(5).1-21

Alharbi, N. S., Alenizi, A. S., Al-Olayan, A. M., Alobaidi, N. A., Algrainy, A. M., Bahadhailah, A. O., Alhunayni, A. A., Alqurashi, H. D., & Alrohaimi, Y. A. (2018). Herbs use in Saudi children with acute respiratory illnesses. *Sudanese Journal of Paediatrics*, *18*(2), 20–24. https://doi.org/10.24911/SJP.106-1538457624

Boadu, A., & Asase, A. (2017). Documentation of herbal medicines used for the treatment and management of human diseases by some communities in southern Ghana. *Evidence-Based Complementary and Alternative Medicine,* Article ID 3043061. https://doi.org/10.1155/2017/3043061

Bodagh, M. N., Maleki, I., & Hekmatdoost, A. (2019). Ginger in gastrointestinal disorders: A systematic review of clinical trials. *Food Science and Nutrition,* *7*(5), 96–108. https://doi.org/10.1002/fsn3.807

Chevallier, A. (2016). *Encyclopedia of herbal medicine: 550 Herbs and remedies for common ailments.* Penguin.

Chumpitazi, B. P., Kearns, G. L., & Shulman, R. J. (2018). Review article: the physiological effects and safety of peppermint oil and its efficacy in irritable bowel syndrome and other functional disorders. *Alimentary Pharmacology & Therapeutics*, *47*(6), 738–752. https://doi.org/10.1111/apt.14519

CMA. (2012). *A–Z Glossary of terms used in herbal medicine.* The Complementary Medical Association. https://www.the-cma.org.uk/Articles/AZ-Glossary-of-Terms-Used-in-Herbal-Medicine-A-3325/

Daniels, E. (2018). 16 Medicinal plants to keep in your home. *ProFlowers.* https://www.proflowers.com/blog/medicinal-plants

Davis, J. (2019). *Harvesting and preserving herbs for the home gardener.* NC State Extension Publication. https://content.ces.ncsu.edu/harvesting-and-preserving-herbs-for-the-home-gardener

Deering, S. (2019). *Nature's 9 most powerful medicinal plants and the science behind them.* Healthline. https://www.healthline.com/

health/most-powerful-medicinal-plants

Easley, T., & Horne, S. (2016). *The modern herbal dispensatory: A medicine-making guide.* North Atlantic Books. ISBN:9781623170806.

Ekor, M. (2014). The growing use of herbal medicines: issues relating to adverse reactions and challenges in monitoring safety. *Frontiers in Pharmacology, 4,* p. 177. https://doi.org/10.3389/fphar.2013.00177

Ellis, M. E. (2020). *Turmeric and other anti-inflammatory spices.* Healthline. https://www.healthline.com/health/osteoarthritis/turmeric-and-anti-inflammatory-herbs#garlic

Fisher, M. Z. (2020). *Steam inhalation: How to use fresh herbs to make your own home remedy for congestion relief.* BusinessInsider. https://www.businessinsider.in/science/health/news/steam-inhalation-how-to-use-fresh-herbs-to-make-your-own-home-remedy-for-congestion-relief/articleshow/78838474.cms

Francis, M. (Undated) Healing herbs: Learn to make infused oils and balms. *HGTV Blogsite.* https://www.hgtv.com/design/make-and-celebrate/handmade/diy-herbal-infused-oils

Frost, R., MacPherson, H., & O'Meara, S. (2013). A critical scoping review of external uses of comfrey (*Symphytum* spp.). *Complementary therapies in medicine, 21*(6), 724–745. https://doi.org/10.1016/j.ctim.2013.09.009

Galan, N. (2019). *8 Herbs and supplements for depression.* Medical News Today. https://www.medicalnewstoday.com/articles/314421

Gardner, D. (2002). Evidence-based decisions about herbal products for treating mental disorders. *Journal of Psychiatry and Neuroscience 27*(5): 324–333. https://www.ncbi.nlm.nih.gov/pmc/articles/PMC161674/

Gartrell, E. (2000). More about the Pond's Collection. Rare Book, Manuscript and Special Collections Library, Duke University. https://library.duke.edu/rubenstein/scriptorium/eaa/ponds.html#note

Ghorbanibirgani, A., Khalili, A., & Zamani, L. (2013). The efficacy of stinging nettle (*Urtica dioica*) in patients with benign prostatic hyperplasia: a randomized double-blind study in 100 patients. *Iranian Red Crescent medical journal, 15*(1), 9–10. https://doi.org/10.5812/ircmj.2386

Gladstar, R. (2014). *Herbs for common ailments – how to make and use herbal remedies for home health care.* Storey Publishing. ISBN: 1612124321, 9781612124322.

GI Society. (2008). Time-tested natural remedies for digestive disorders. Canadian Society of Intestinal Research. First published in the *Inside Tract newsletter 165.* https://badgut.org/information-centre/a-z-digestive-topics/time-tested-natural-remedies-for-digestive-disorders/

Hewlings, S. J., & Kalman, D. S. (2017). Curcumin: A review of its effects on human health. *Foods (Basel, Switzerland)*, 6(10), 92. https://doi.org/10.3390/foods6100092

Huizen, J. (2020). *Home and natural remedies for upset stomach.* Medical News Today. https://www.medicalnewstoday.com/articles/322047

Iwanaga, M., Iwanaga, H., Kawakami, N., & World Mental Health Japan Survey Group (2017). Twelve-month use of herbal medicines as a remedy for mental health problems in Japan: A cross-national analysis of World Mental Health Survey data. *Asia-Pacific Psychiatry* 9(3), https://doi.org/10.1111/appy.12285

Jeanroy, E. (2019). How to make herbal infusions. *The Spruce Eats Blogsite.* https://www.thespruceeats.com/how-to-make-an-herbal-infusion-1762142

Johns Cupp, M. (1999). Herbal remedies: Adverse effects and drug interactions. *American Family Physician* 59(5), 1239-1244. https://www.aafp.org/afp/1999/0301/p1239.html

Johnson, T. (2020). *11 Supplements for Menopause.* WebMD. https://www.webmd.com/menopause/ss/slideshow-menopause

Kaur, J., Kaur, S., & Mahajan, A. (2013). Herbal medicine: Possible risks and benefits. *American Journal of Phytomedicine and Clinical Therapeutics* 1(2), 226–239. https://www.imedpub.com/articles/herbal-medicines-possible-risks-andbenefits.pdf

Keiley, L. (2006). *6 Natural Allergy Remedies.* Mother Earth News. https://www.motherearthnews.com/natural-health/natural-allergy-remedies-zmaz06aszraw

Kyrou, I., Christou, A., Panagiotakos, D., Stefanaki, C., Skenderi, K., Katsana, K., & Tsigos, C. (2017). Effects of a hops (*Humulus lupulus* L.) dry extract supplement on self-reported depression, anxiety and stress levels in apparently healthy young adults: A randomized, placebo-controlled, double-blind, crossover pilot study. *Hormones (Athens, Greece)*, 16(2), 171–180. https://doi.org/10.14310/horm.2002.1738

Liang, W., Xu, W., Zhu, J., Zhu, Y., Gu, Q., Li, Y., Guo, C., Huang, Y., Yu, J., Wang, W., Hu, Y., Zhao, Y., Han, B., Bei, W., & Guo, J. (2020). *Ginkgo biloba* extract improves brain uptake of ginsenosides by increasing blood-brain barrier permeability via activating A1 adenosine receptor signaling pathway. *Journal of Ethnopharmacology*, 246, 112243. https://doi.org/10.1016/j.jep.2019.112243

Lu, X., Samuelson, D. R., Rasco, B. A., & Konkel, M. E.

(2012). Antimicrobial effect of diallyl sulphide on *Campylobacter jejuni* biofilms. *Journal of Antimicrobial Chemotherapy*, 67(8), 1915–1926. https://doi.org/10.1093/jac/dks138

Massoud, A., El Sisi, S., Salama, O., & Massoud, A. (2001) Preliminary study of therapeutic efficacy of a new fasciolicidal drug derived from *Commiphora molmol* (myrrh). *The American Journal of Tropical Medicine and Hygiene*, 65(2), 96–99. https://doi.org/10.4269/ajtmh.2001.65.96

Motaleb, M. A., Hossain, M. K., Sobhan, I., Alam, M. K., Khan N. A., & Firoz, R. (2011) *Selected medicinal plants of Chittagong Hill tracts*. IUCN, Dhaka, Bangladesh. https://www.iucn.org/content/selected-medicinal-plants-chittagong-hill-tracts

Mulrow, C., Lawrence, V., Jacobs, B., Dennehy, C., Sapp, J. Ramirez, G., Aguilar, C., Montgomery, K., Morbidoni, L. Arterburn, J. M., Chiquette, E., Harris, M., Mullins, D., Vickers, A., & Flora, K. (2000). Milk thistle: Effects on liver disease and cirrhosis and clinical adverse effects; Summary. *AHRQ Evidence Report Summaries*, 21. Rockville (MD): Agency for Healthcare Research and Quality (US); 1998-2005. https://www.ncbi.nlm.nih.gov/books/NBK11896/

Petrovska, B. (2012). Historical review of medicinal plants' usage. *Pharmacognosy Reviews*, 6(11), 1–5. https://doi.org/10.4103/0973-7847.95849

Pittler, M. H., & Ernst, E. (2004). Feverfew for preventing migraine. *The Cochrane Database of Systematic Reviews*, (1), CD002286. https://doi.org/10.1002/14651858.CD002286.pub2

Ratini, M. (2019). *Natural cold and flu remedies*. WebMD. https://www.webmd.com/cold-and-flu/ss/slideshow-natural-cold-and-flu-remedies

Salleh, A. (2014). *Plant chemicals could help Alzheimer's*. ABC Science. URL: https://www.abc.net.au/science/articles/2014/10/15/4098476.htm

Setright, R. (2017). Prevention of symptoms of gastric irritation (GERD) using two herbal formulas: An observational study. *Journal of the Australian Traditional-Medicine Society*, 23(2), 68–71. https://search.informit.org/doi/10.3316/informit.950298610899394 (Original work published June 2017)

Shah, S. A., Sander, S., White, C. M., Rinaldi, M., & Coleman, C. I. (2007). Evaluation of echinacea for the prevention and treatment of the common cold: a meta-analysis. *The Lancet Review*, 7(7), 473–480. https://doi.org/10.1016/S1473-3099(07)70160-3

Shiel, W. Jr. (Undated). *Herbs: Toxicities and drug interactions*. MedicineNet. https://www.medicinenet.com/herbs___toxicities_

and_drug_interactions/views.htm

Schrum, C. (2018). *13 Natural remedies for common ailments.* ExperienceLife. https://experiencelife.com/article/13-natural-remedies-for-common-ailments/

Tabassum, N. & Ahmad, F. (2011) Role of natural herbs in the treatment of hypertension. *Pharmacognosy Review 5*(9), pp. 30–40. https://doi.org/10.4103/0973-7847.79097 https://www.ncbi.nlm.nih.gov/pmc/articles/PMC3210006/

Vickers, A., Zollman, C., & Lee, R. (2001). Herbal medicine. *The Western Journal of Medicine, 175*(2), 125–128. https://doi.org/10.1136/ewjm.175.2.125

Widrig, R., Suter, A., Saller, R., & Melzer, J. (2007). Choosing between NSAID and arnica for topical treatment of hand osteoarthritis in a randomised, double-blind study. *Rheumatology International, 27,* 585–591. https://doi.org/10.1007/s00296-007-0304-y

Wikipedia. (2020). *History of herbalism.* Wikipedia. https://en.wikipedia.org/wiki/History_of_herbalism

Wikipedia. (2021). *Medicinal plants.* Wikipedia. https://en.wikipedia.org/wiki/Medicinal_plants

Wolff, H. H., & Kieser, M. (2007). Hamamelis in children with skin disorders and skin injuries: Results of an observational study. *European Journal of Pediatrics, 166*(9), 943–948. https://doi.org/10.1007/s00431-006-0363-1

Wills, R. B. H., Bone, K. & Morgan, M. (2000). Herbal products: Active constituents, modes of action, and quality control. *Nutrition Research Reviews 13,* pp. 47–77. https://www.cambridge.org/core/services/aop-cambridge-core/content/view/8E5D4F8734D795BB107F89E6E5CB8587/S0954422400000044a.pdf/div-class-title-herbal-products-active-constituents-modes-of-action-and-quality-control-div.pdf

Wu, M., Liu, L., Xing, Y., Yang, S., Li, H., & Cao, Y. (2020). Roles and mechanisms of hawthorn and its extracts on atherosclerosis: A review. *Frontiers in Pharmacology, 11,* 118. https://doi.org/10.3389/fphar.2020.00118

Zhang, J., Onakpoya, I. J., Posadzki, P., & Eddouks, M. (2015). The safety of herbal medicine: From prejudice to evidence. *Evidence-Based Complementary and Alternative Medicine,* Article ID 316706. https://doi.org/10.1155/2015/316706

Zick, S. M., Schwabl, H., Flower, A., Chakraborty, B., & Hirschkorn, K. (2009). Unique aspects of herbal whole system research. *Explore (New York), 5*(2), 97–103. https://doi.org/10.1016/j.explore.2008.12.001

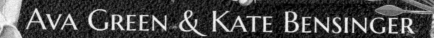

Ava Green & Kate Bensinger

GROW
YOUR OWN
MEDICINE

HANDBOOK FOR THE
SELF-SUFFICIENT HERBALIST

Library of Congress Control Number: 2021952743

Important notice

Please note the information contained within this document is for educational and entertainment purposes only. The book is written by experienced and knowledgeable herbalism enthusiasts, not physicians. No parts of this book are meant to replace the advice of a medical professional. Do not try self-diagnosis or attempt self-treatment for serious or long-term problems without first consulting a qualified medical herbalist or medical practitioner as appropriate. Do not take any herb without first referring to the safety sections and always check with your physician. Do not exceed any dosages recommended. Always consult a professional practitioner if symptoms persist. If taking prescribed medicines, seek professional medical advice before using herbal remedies. Take care to correctly identify plants and do not harvest restricted or banned species. The Publisher and the author make no representations or warranties with respect to the accuracy or completeness of the contents of this work and specifically disclaim all warranties, including without limitation warranties of fitness for a particular purpose.

Practice, laws, and regulations all change, and the reader should obtain up-to-date professional advice on any such issues. You should research your local laws before using the information in this book. The authors and the publisher expressly disclaim any liability, loss, or risk, personal or otherwise, which is incurred as a consequence, directly or indirectly, of the use and application of any of the contents of this book.

The authors are not your healthcare providers. This book is a beginner-friendly guide, free of heavy and complex terminology, offering a simple and step-by-step approach to herbalism.

This book provides content related to physical and/or mental health issues. As such, use of this book implies your acceptance of this disclaimer.

Special Bonus!

Join Our FB group to find new herbal recipes and to share experiences with your new herbal friends!

Scan this QR code below to get the LINK to our FB group! See you there!

www.theherb.space/group

Contents

Herb List

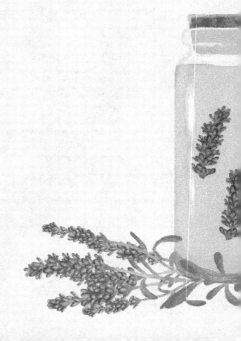

Introduction

Ever wonder where that veggie, fruit, or herb came from? What chemicals were used to grow it? Is it healthy or even safe? What about that expensive medicine you took not so long ago, when you weren't feeling so well?

There is an unlimited number of plants around us, to be used for food and medicine, for FREE! And we don't even know they exist. Some are not discovered yet ... Strangely, we rely solely on conventional medicine to treat our ailments – well, not all of us, but many. Allopathic medicine has its place ONLY when we are not able to cure ourselves with lighter and friendlier natural medicine that has been available to us through thousands of years.

But, where do you start? Whom do you trust to be your guide? Where do you find out about which herbs to grow and how to grow them? How do you choose which herbs to use? You don't even have a backyard ... oh, my goodness, so many unanswered questions, right?

But, that's about to change. For you, my lovely reader, I will be the guide you need in order to become self-sufficient and grow (almost) everything you require, whether you live in a beautiful country house or a modern apartment. Don't you worry. I will start with some fun herbal history, and I will talk about the basics of any garden. Then I will show you, depending on your location and living situation, what can be suitable for YOU. Every garden is unique and I will show you how I easily turned my friends into lifelong herbalists; by the end of this book, you might become one too. I will also show you some 50 different plants that you can grow, as well as describe what problems can arise and HOW to deal with them. I've got you covered.

My life has always been filled with the wonders of herbs. I distinctly remember the sweet scent of chamomile to help me fall asleep during bedtime stories. I still smell the wafts of lavender that tickled my nose as I passed by my nana's room. During the cold winters, the dance of ginger and garlic filled the house and bites of paprika and turmeric fought off debilitating colds and flu. I remember my nana, with her large straw hat shielding her face from the afternoon sun. She spent hours each day in the garden, planting, pruning, and tending to each plant. But what I remember most, is the wealth of knowledge she shared with me about those precious plants. She also gave me small tasks to do; Nana paid me a nickel for every hornworm I found and removed from the tomatoes. I discovered the world of herbs when growing plants was popular in the late 60s. I wasn't satisfied with 'just' a house plant; mine had to DO something. I started with a few herbs, mostly inside the house. Nana taught me about the earth, the richness and bounty of the soil beneath our feet. She taught me the secrets of all the plants that she knew, and she taught me about the independence that they provide us.

Perhaps this is the reason that I have never looked at herbal remedies and alternative methods of healing through plants as strange. My life never gave me a reason to be skeptical, for I have only grown up with the phenomenal benefits that herbalism offers.

My herbal journey really started with a rose geranium. Mom and I visited every greenhouse in a 50-mile radius and finally found one that stocked this old-fashioned plant. When we arrived, I discovered they also carried a trove of botanicals: 15 different scented geraniums, seven different kinds of true mints, ten varieties of thyme, three types of sage, and so much more. Mom indulged my passion for plants and allowed me to spend $50, a hefty sum for a teen to spend in 1970. I delighted in researching my herbs and finding out how to grow them successfully. Best of all, I sold my bounty of herbs to fund my new-found hobby.

Ever since that day, I have continued to learn, grow, and share my knowledge about herbs. I have discovered many of the culinary, medicinal, scent, dye, and decorative purposes of the plants all around us. Medicinal herbs became my specialty and I've grown over 183 different types of herbs.

During my lifetime, I have trained as a nurse and a self-taught herbalist. I consumed every bit of information

I could find in books at the library. I attended lectures by many of the greats, like Dr. James Duke, Michael Tierra, Billy Joe Tatum, LaDean Griffin, Susan Weed, Dr. John Christopher, Rosemary Gladstar, and others. Finally, in 2002, I received a degree in Naturopathy with Herbal Emphasis, and felt that the studies had filled the gaps in my knowledge. Everyday I continue practicing and learning.

In this book, I strive to provide you with the wisdom and power of healing that is found naturally from the earth. This is knowledge that should be accessible to everyone. Self-healing is a power that you can have, once you learn the correct methods of planting, growing, caring, and harvesting.

Reading this book will guide you through the steps you need to take to be a successful herb gardener. I can assure you that, after starting your herbalism journey, you will save your money and your health. The minimal cost of building an herb garden saves you ten-fold on pharmaceuticals, flavoring and cleaning supplies that you would otherwise purchase throughout your life. You will always have just what you need on hand, even in the middle of the night. If your child wakes up at 4am with a stomach ache, you'll feel at ease knowing that you won't have to wait until the pharmacy opens to help them find relief. Your herb garden will become one of the most rewarding and fun-filled hobbies. That's the power of our connection with nature. And you'll feel deeply satisfied and confident knowing that you have the knowledge to help yourself and your family and no one can take that away from you.

Dozens of people have thanked me for helping them design and grow the flourishing herb gardens that have changed their lives ... and in this book I will show you exactly what I taught them.

With my guidance, your determination, and the patience to learn, you will be equipped with the skills to grow the herbs you need. You'll be able to make delicious meals and clean your house without using commercial poisons. Best of all, you'll have natural medicines on hand to prevent and relieve illnesses without running to the drugstore. You'll have the herbs for a dream home apothecary.

Preventing or treating a disease in its early stages leads to more success with greater ease. The sooner you start absorbing the positive energy of your garden and the essence of its medicines, the better. Your herb garden will provide a sense of pride that comes from fortifying your own health. It's crucial for you to take action now for a healthier and happier life.

The methods you will learn in this book are proven to yield incredible results with herb gardens, of all sizes and shapes, in any home. By following the guidelines in this book, you will succeed at growing an herb garden that eliminates your need to run to the pharmacy and reduces grocery store purchases.

This book is not a one and done read. It is a manual filled with decades of herbal knowledge and wisdom. I hope that this book becomes your mentor, the way my nana was to me. This book is my way of honoring her wisdom, and the wisdom of all the herbalists who have gifted us this powerful knowledge. May we always use it wisely and share this wisdom with everyone we meet along our journeys. So what are you waiting for? Let's dive into your herbalism journey!

Why Do You Need an Herb Garden?

Self-empowerment, self-worth, peace of mind and greater financial independence are all reasons to begin an herb garden. I was astonished that, before they started their own herb gardens, my friends were spending just under what the average American spends on over-the-counter medicine, which was roughly around $900 per year. That money has now gone into savings, house renovations and even vacations. It may not sound like a lot, but when you add up the bills, that mole hill turns into a mountain.

Cooking is probably what you think of first when you hear the word 'herbs' but that's not the whole picture. While cooking with herbs has added much flavor to my diet and has allowed me to reduce salt use, herbs can be used for so much more. Herbal decorations add beauty and fragrance to my home. I make many of my own skin care products. This allows me to avoid unwanted ingredients. The medicinal use of herbs, though, is honestly the most impressive aspect of herbs for me, and that is what brings me to you now.

Why Grow Your Own Herbs?

An herb garden most certainly has a startup cost, but you can start slowly. I recommend starting with the research, planning and preparation, before diving into planting. Doing that will help you cut costs wherever you can and make the most out of the area you have available.

It's not necessary to be an artist to create an appealing yet useful environment around your home. Many herbs are attractive and can be planted in flower or curbside gardens. The weedier-looking plants you may wish to grow in a location towards the back of the garden, hidden by the presence of prettier herbs in front of them. Or you could grow them in the backyard where appearance won't matter. But you may find, like I did, that even the homeliest plants can produce some really beautiful flowers.

I have brought this book to you to empower you to take your health into your own hands, to find your happiness and inspiration in the garden, and really to thrive in every way – body, mind, and soul. I want the world to experience the abundance of the earth in the same way that I and so many others have. Before we jump into the herb garden itself, and all the great medicinal, culinary, and decorative herbs that you can have at your doorstep, let us look at the benefits of herbalism throughout the world.

Benefits of Herbalism

In my own life I can't imagine my days without the presence of herbs, or what my life would be if I had to rely on pharmacies or doctors for all medications. Medicine has come to the point that we cannot avoid its use in modern healthcare. However, to not see the benefits of herbal medicine in your daily life is to miss out on a lot. I know that herbalism has always been a part of my life and I would like to discuss a few of the exceptional benefits overall, as well as those that fit into daily life.

Herbalism really saves me money and I am sure that saving money is something everyone would love to do. Learning about herbs and growing them will most certainly help with that. As I mentioned before, I don't need to run to the store for seasoning for a dish, or purchase something to soften my skin, or relieve an illness.

I do have a routine doctor's checkup, but that is about it. I am blessed to have my health in tip-top shape, but I attribute that to Mother Earth's bounty. I rely on Mother Earth for everything. There is not a conventional headache pill in my house, nor any pills for nausea, or any other common medicine normally found in households. The herbs are my medicine cabinet.

Not only does an herbal garden save you money, but it also saves you time. It empowers you to be the master of your own body and health.

It truly has increased my sense of wellbeing. I feel more energetic than most people my age. The garden is not only my physical medicine but also my soul medicine. Modern life has become very stressful, yet there is nothing on earth as rejuvenating and relaxing as planting and harvesting from the garden.

Gardening is a very interesting physical activity. I find it much more enjoyable than going to the gym! Gardening can be adjusted to as much or as little as you are able to do. For example, my first garden was fairly large and in the ground. My next, however, was small and mostly consisted of raised beds, due to time constraints that had developed in my life. Beds can be raised to counter height to allow those in a wheelchair, or those who find it hard to get up and down a lot, to garden. A dear elderly friend of mine was so happy to discover she could continue gardening in raised beds, even after her arthritis made it nearly impossible to do it the traditional way. All the different scents and textures involved can appeal especially to blind people. Herb gardens really are fully customizable to fit your needs.

Growing your own herbs also means you know exactly where they come from. In this increasingly toxic world, this is a great comfort. You will know all the details about how your plants were grown and what chemicals were (or were not) used on them. Not a day goes by when there's not some story circulating in the media about recalls on food items, GMOs, or lawsuits due to chemicals. In this way you can help nature repair the earth. We owe it to Mother Nature to respect and help her, as all life depends on this world. We are a part of everything, after all. It may be a small part, but together we can do much harm. The good news, however, is that we can also do much good.

Pharmaceutical medicines have so many side effects that destroy our bodies. The medicines are usually not 100% safe and normally only treat the symptoms and not the root causes. In addition, they potentially cause more problems, which are then treated with

more medicine. The ugly cycle only continues from there. I have seen this first hand from a medication that a friend was taking. It helped the initial issue but then caused unbearable nausea. The doctors gave her medicine for that but it caused chronic headaches. After all that, they had to start over. The discomfort she endured was terrible and unnecessary.

Herbs are different: they have a whole-body effect when you use them, and they heal exactly where healing is needed, without the many unwanted side effects. Of course, we must understand that what can do good can also cause harm if not used properly. This is why it's important to understand the herb before using it. However, once you get the hang of it, once you have the knowledge, there is no end to the empowerment of your life through using herbs. Herbalism has never left us. It's only become more efficient and better studied. Let us look at the history of the use of herbs through the ages.

The Mysterious History of Herbal Medicine

Herbs – plants used for culinary, medicinal, color/decorative and scent purposes – have a fascinating history and an amazing diversity of uses. Humans have been using herbs to improve life for thousands of years – for longer even than written history.

The journey has been a long one, stretching all the way back to the Neanderthals. The Neanderthals existed on earth from around 430,000 years

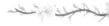

ago and disappeared altogether around 30,000 years ago. We believed they were predominately meat-eaters, but evidence in the 21st century has shown us that they were knowledgeable in using plants such as yarrow, willow, and St. John's wort (Hardy et al., 2012).

Our studies have shown that the medicinal use of herbs stretches as far back as 60,000 years ago in Iraq. A recipe found in Mesopotamia was dated to 1730 BCE and is the oldest written example of culinary use. The oldest known record of the intentional use of herbs to repel insects was found in South Africa and dated at 77, 000 years ago. We also know that herbal medicine used by African people is the oldest (Mahomoodally, 2013), but least documented, even today. Herbal medicine among the Native American people also stretches many thousands of years back, but isn't as well documented as we would like. However, we know of the incredible medicine from Native Americans and others, such as the Aboriginal people of Australia, through word of mouth. This is also seen in Iran, India, China and pretty much the rest of the world as well. Today, we have little knowledge unless we are born into the

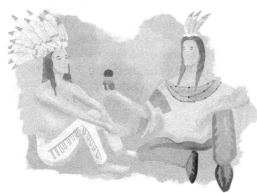

tradition. I believe I was just lucky to be born into a family of herbal wise ones and to be able to continue the passing on of this valuable knowledge.

Since the beginning of humanity, we have had herbalism. To further

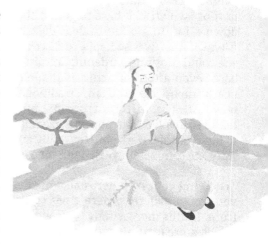

understand this movement of medicine throughout the ages, we need to look at the history of the written records.

We attribute the earliest known records of herbal medicine to the Rig Veda (2500 BCE), an ancient Indian collection of Sanskrit hymns. In the Rig Veda, this entry explains the reverence that people had toward the plant kingdom and its medicine (Gupta, 2013):

*"You herbs, born at the birth of time
More ancient than the gods themselves.
O Plants, with this hymn I sing to you
Our mothers and our gods."*

From these dates, we move along our journey to find that, across the Mesopotamian world, people praised herbal medicine highly. Just like with the Chinese, the written texts of medicinal herb usage represented documentations of millennia of wisdom. The oldest known Mesopotamian text is a medical therapeutic text that came out of the Ur III period (2112–2004 BCE) (Scurlock & Andersen, 2005). The Ebers Papyrus is the next text to emerge (1550 BCE) and, 1,000 years later, we find evidence of the use of herbal tinctures, creams and oils in Persia, which is modern-day Iran.

While much of the medicine around

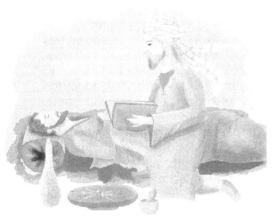

the world remained almost stagnant in its approach, it was the medicine of Greece and the work of Hippocrates, 'The Father of Medicine,' that was the basis for modern medicine. Hippocrates concentrated on around 250 of the native plants on the Greek island of Kos. Even though he did not formally describe the plants, it is said that the locals have no problem identifying them (Fanouriou et al., 2018).

Herbalism spread across the entire world, growing in depth at different speeds. If we look at the vast Celtic knowledge of herbalism, we see how it dominated Central and Western Europe between 800 BCE and 500 CE. Yet the wisdom is only documented in a few manuscripts, such as the four known as the 'Meddygon Myddfai,' which were compiled and published in 1861 by John Pughe.

When Christopher Columbus first landed in the Americas he sent many herbs, used by the indigenous people, back to Spain, where they were added to the European herbs.

Europeans making their way to North America carried seeds and plants with them into the great unknown to ensure they had access to familiar herbs. The fact that space was severely limited on the transport ships, yet the colonists still chose to carry plants with them, showed how important these plants were.

There isn't a culture that has not experienced some form of herbal food and medicine. The Inuit people were nomadic and they still used herbal medicines, and attributed healing benefits to plants (Qitsualik, 2021).

For a while, naturopathic and allopathic medicine were equals in English speaking countries, each with colleges of medicine. The introduction of synthetic drugs and the fact they were patentable, and therefore economically profitable, led to a decline in the use of herbs for health, and a preference for allopathic medicine.

Inspired by the back-to-the land movement, a general dissatisfaction with modern medicine, and a preference for prevention instead of waiting for something to break, there started a revival in the use of herbs. Today, our culture is experiencing a blending of the best of both natural and allopathic medicine.

Our Responsibility to Mother Earth

Every human being has ancestors or relatives belonging to an indigenous society. Regardless of our cultural origins, we all have a sacred responsibility to look after the Earth. We need to respect and look after our home. After all, where would any of us be without it?

The first rule of respect is to do no harm. In the wild, never harvest more than one plant in ten. Even if a plant is plentiful locally, it may be endangered overall. If you harvest one-tenth and somebody else harvests one-tenth, and somebody else harvests one-tenth, they all add up to about a third of the total population. When harvesting from one plant, even your own, only harvest up to a third of the plant to ensure the plant stays healthy and can continue growing properly. Growing your own helps protect endangered herbs from overexploitation.

Another way to help is to control those plants that may become invasive. Harvesting properly prevents ripening of seeds for many herbs, but not for all, and sometimes you wish to have seeds. The wind or animals such as birds, chipmunks, and even the fur of larger animals can carry seed very far from home. To prevent plants from becoming invasive, when an herb seed is ripening, collect it and place it thoughtfully where it won't be able to spread and cause problems.

Be careful what you put on and in the land. Many chemicals persist for a very long time and are poisonous to all life. My people believe in venerating the Earth and caring for her. We believe that we are the caretakers of this Earth. This should apply not only to my people, but to every person on this planet and to those who come after us. By looking after her, she looks after us. She provides us with food, medicine and, of course, our beautiful home.

It is not only we who need the plants for food and medicine, but all the animals as well. When we look after the flora, we are naturally taking care of the animals too.

My people believe in balance. My grandmother always told me about balance, and how it was our responsibility to keep it. Never take anything without giving back and always give thanks for the gifts of the Earth. Always remember to walk in the balance.

Discovering the Foundations of Your Wonder Garden

Each time that I guide a friend or a client through the beginning stages of gardening, the first reaction leaves a little sweat on his or her brow. I empathize with them and tell them not to worry; that soon they will be the master. It seems like a lot of information at first, especially the foundations that a beginner gardener needs to know; it certainly was for me. But once you have done everything, just once, believe me, it only gets easier. No one honestly believes me when I tell them it gets easier, until they find themselves teaching others. This is the moment that I find the most beautiful: when people have that special glint in their eyes and gardening becomes the best medicine on earth. You too will be there soon, trust me.

Soil

As you can guess, your soil is the most important part of your gardening process. Whether you choose to be an indoor or outdoor gardener, the quality of your soil determines the quality of the plants you can grow. Your soil consists of different layers and is not just one layer of everything, all squished together. How you go about preparing your soil is important because of these layers.

The soil actually consists of three layers. The first and top layer is your topsoil. This layer can always be improved and changed by adding more organic matter, sand, and such. It is important to know that this layer is where you find your fungi, earthworms, insects and bacteria. The web of life lives here and disturbing it all the time is never a good idea. The second layer is your subsoil, this layer has the purpose of either being good or bad for drainage. Below that is what is known as the parent rock, this is the place where your soil was 'born.' It happens over millennia, and it is a slow process whereby the rock gets broken down into smaller pieces. It is good to know what your parent rock is because it dictates the normal consistency of the soil.

Topsoil

The best topsoil contains a mixture of clay, sand, and organic humus. In reality, very little topsoil is perfect. Most places naturally tend to one type or the other.

This is my experience, unfortunately. Where I live, the dirt is acidic clay with gravel for drainage and it makes growing things difficult without extra effort.

Humus

Humus is the dark organic matter that forms in soil when dead plants and animal matter (including compost and mulch) are broken down.

Humus has many nutrients, nitrogen being the most important. It is difficult to define humus because it is complex and not fully understood. It differs from compost both in the size of particles and the organisms doing the breaking down; humus organisms are anaerobic (require an absence of oxygen), whereas organisms that break down compost are aerobic (require oxygen).

Soils that have a healthy mixture will have a humus content of 8–10%.

Clay Soil

Clay is a fine-grained, natural mineral in soil. Clay soil is very elastic when wet but is hard and cracks when it is dry. It is usually acidic but very fertile, once the pH is adjusted.

Clay soil drains water slowly. The soil around a house is often a clay subsoil, excavated when the house was built. Flower beds around the house are often different from the rest of the yard. They need improvement in order to ensure good plant growth.

My current yard naturally has clay-type soil and is very acidic. At first I added lime at the rate indicated by my soil test, but subsequent years of adding compost has lightened and sweetened my topsoil. I used to say that if it weren't for the gravel, I'd have no drainage. I have removed much of that gravel as I slowly amended the soil in my gardens.

Sand

The tiny pieces of rock or shell that make up sand are what give it its attractive color. Different places have different types of sand due to the variety of rock and shell available there. Sandy soil is easy to determine by its feel. It has a gritty texture and when a handful of sandy soil is squeezed, it will quickly fall apart when you open your hand. Soil that is predominantly sand drains very fast and many nutrients leach out every time you water or it rains.

Gravelly soil has great drainage but grows crooked roots and is often hard to dig in. Don't remove the gravel without providing for drainage in another way.

Good soil is well drained but retains enough moisture for the plants grown in it. There are many nifty tools on the market that test the moisture content of your soil, but gauging this might seem difficult without the top notch tools. It really isn't that difficult at all. My grandmother used to make me grab clumps of soil from different areas of the garden. Then I'd run and show her. Sometimes she would tell me to go and water this side, and sometimes the other side. I didn't understand what all this was about, but it was fun nonetheless. What she was teaching me was how to test the moisture level of the soil.

When you go into the garden, pick up a sample of the top layer of soil. Place this into one of your hands and form a ball. Squeeze it tight. When you open your hand, one of three things can happen. The ball can completely fall apart out of your hand, which means that your soil is far too sandy and/or dry. If the ball becomes a lump of clay, leaving water on your hands, this means it's far too wet. When the ball stays firm in your hand but there is no moisture coming off on your hand, you have got the perfect amount of moisture in your soil.

Just like my grandmother taught me, make sure to check a few different areas in the garden, and not just one spot. Make sure the soil is just right all the way around the garden. If it isn't, adjust it and retest.

Light

Light allows your herbs to make food for themselves, through photosynthesis. While most of us might not remember what we were taught about this process in science class at school, it's enough to know that sunlight on a plant's leaves causes a chemical reaction unique to plants. All of life on earth depends on the fact that plants can make food in this way.

I learned to grow herbs in partial shade when I lived where the sun was strong. Many herbs grown outside will reward you when given a little shady protection during the heat of the day.

Inside, you can rely on the sun through a window but it's often not strong enough. My first efforts resulted in leggy plants that leaned towards the light. Many got weaker as the winter went on and the sunlight became less intense. While that doesn't happen everywhere, I needed artificial light to supplement the sunlight in that locality.

Fluorescent or LED shop lights induce vegetative growth, including early herb starts, just fine. Flowers and fruit (reproductive growth) require the ultraviolet spectrum of light which is filtered out by glass, often added to old-fashioned greenhouses that don't have fiberglass roofs. Grow bulbs or tubes provide that extra spectrum.

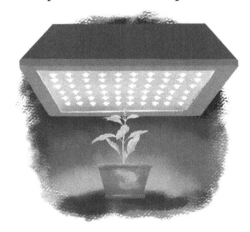

Potting Mix

Sterile potting mix is best for starting plants that will later be transplanted into bigger pots or the garden. It drains well yet will hold nutrients. The very conditions that promote seed germination also promote the growth of diseases. While I'll tell you how to deal with them in their own chapter, the use of sterile soil will mean that your herbs won't have to face those issues until they are bigger. After your herbs are big enough to see, add a half strength fertilizer, such as compost or nettle tea or an organic commercial fertilizer. If you have more than a few pots, it's much cheaper to mix up your own soil. This will also allow you to customize the mix to meet different needs.

DIY Potting Mix

1 part coconut coir or peat
½ part perlite, vermiculite
½ part pine bark or sand
½ part screened compost

Mix together thoroughly. Dampen and sterilize to use for starting seedlings (how-to guide below). Does not need to be sterilized to fill pots for established plants. If a 10 quart bucket is used as the measure for 1 part, the finished mix will fill five 12 inch (30 cm) pots.

How to Sterilize Small Amounts of Soil

Heating soil to 180°F (82°C) will kill weed seeds and most pathogens. You can do very small amounts in a pressure cooker, bake them in your oven, or use your microwave. Using the first two methods will make your house odoriferous (i.e., stinky) so I recommend using the microwave method. In fact I bought a used one at a yard sale for that very purpose. Below are the easy steps.

1. Place the soil to be sterilized in a plastic trash bag. Do not fill it more than one-third full.

2. Dampen the soil. Do not make it soggy, just moist.

3. Close the top of the bag, pressing out all the air as you do. Tie it firmly shut. I just tie the top in an overhand knot. You want it tight so the steam from a later step can't escape.

4. Place the whole thing in your microwave and heat it. The time of heating will depend on how much soil you put in it. When you have heated it enough, the bag will blow up like a balloon from the steam formed.

5. Next, and this is important, cool the whole bag before opening it.

6. Once cool, open and use or store in the bag.

Water

Water is the next important factor needed for your herbs. Too dry and they wilt and die. Too wet and, unless they're a swamp plant, they'll rot and die. The trick is to provide just enough. It is easy to give too much or too little water, so it is important to know the needs of each particular plant.

Most young plants need regular watering until they're well rooted. Once well established though, most are slightly drought resistant. Be careful not to over-water. One quick and common way to test the moisture is to stick your finger into the soil up to the second knuckle. All is well if you feel dampness. If dry, you need to water. There are also several types of water meters available in gardening centers and catalogs, if you're inclined to gadgets. I much prefer to test it myself using the finger method as I feel it provides a more accurate reading and really helps connect me more with my plants and the whole process of growing them.

One important tip is to water the soil, not your herbs. That keeps the water off their leaves to help control diseases and prevent sunburn. A leaky hose or drip irrigation can really help. Leaky hoses are affordable and I strongly recommend their use if your garden bed is large. If you're growing in pots, water from the bottom and never leave water in the saucer for longer than an hour as that will encourage root rot.

Make sure your water isn't working against you. Chlorine and other chemicals are added to city water to prevent the growth of algae, bacteria and other life. A little won't hurt, but too much of it will harm your plants, particularly if you have to water often. Filling a bucket or water barrel and letting the water sit overnight will allow it to offgas. This is a simple and inexpensive way to protect your plants. Mulch and compost can also provide much protection to your outdoor plants. Filter if you have to. If you feel it's necessary to test your water for harmful chemicals, you can get test strips at most home and garden stores as well as at hardware stores.

Feeding Your Garden

Plants are rooted to one spot, whether in the ground, in a raised bed, or in a container. You must go to them to provide the food and water they need. On the other hand, they can't run away so if they don't get what they need from you, they suffer and ultimately die. I can't tell you the number of plants I accidentally murdered in the beginning because I didn't know much about feeding them. Whoops.

There are many organic fertilizers on the market. Compost is available in bags to purchase. Fertilizer is measured by NPK levels, the most important chemicals to your herbs.

N stands for nitrogen. Nitrogen is needed by plants in order to produce chlorophyll, the green pigment that can trap energy from sunlight. Without chlorophyll, a plant's leaves will be yellow and it won't be able to make food, so its growth will be stunted. But the role of nitrogen is more complex than that.

Once I grew great pot marigold plants. The green, leafy plants were beautiful but they didn't bloom until very late in the season. I had given up hope by then! When I asked my grandmother what was wrong, thinking it was the seed or something, she said I had provided too much nitrogen. It seems that excess nitrogen stimulates vegetative growth at the expense of flowers and fruit.

Natural sources of nitrogen you can use include bone meal, blood meal, or fish emulsion (a quick-acting organic liquid fertilizer made from byproducts of the fish oil and fish meal industry). Another option, and my personal favorite, is that you can plant a legume cover crop, such as clover or fenugreek. Legumes have symbiotic bacteria in root nodules that fix nitrogen from the air and thereby enrich the soil with this element.

P stands for phosphorus. This element is usually sourced from green manure crops, manure, bone meal, crab and shrimp waste, and phosphate rocks. It is not usually an issue but a lack of phosphorus can cause diminished plant growth, reduced crop yield, and a delay in plant maturity. Potassium is much more important.

K is for potassium (how random, right?!). It is often called pot-ash from an early source – hardwood ash. Wood ash is an excellent source of both lime and potassium. Not only that, but using ashes in the garden also provides many of the trace elements that plants need to thrive. But ash is best used either lightly scattered, or by first being composted as an ingredient in your pile. Wood ash will produce lye when it gets wet. In small quantities, this lye will not cause problems, but in larger amounts, the lye may burn your plants.

Compost

Compost is the best overall fertilizer to feed your herbs as well as to add organic matter to your garden. Compost contains the basic NPK, but also has many trace minerals that make your plants healthy and more resistant to pests and diseases. My thrifty grandmother taught me to make my own compost, turning food scraps and yard waste into this black gold. Compost can cure many ills. If your soil is mostly clay, add organic matter. If your soil is too sandy, add organic matter. Worn out soil is also improved by ... you guessed it ... adding compost. Compost is basically plant matter that has been digested by bacteria and incorporated into soil. It provides fertilizer and contains many minerals and trace minerals important for healthy plant growth. The best compost is made of 3 parts brown and one part green matter and must heat up to at least 160°F (70°C). I can't wait to tell you all about composting and how I make my mine for free in the 'Becoming the

Guardian Angel of Your Garden' chapter.

I feed my plants, but not too much, and I water my herbs, but not too much. Too much fertilizer will weaken the natural oils and other constituents that make herbs so valuable. These natural constituents evolved in plants to protect them against insects, sun and disease and to attract pollinators. But they are also valued for their flavor, scent, dye, medicinal and nutritional properties. Plants that had to work hard to survive tend to build these chemicals up. This makes them stronger than plants that have had things easy. An herb gardener's job is to find balance between giving too much and not enough resources to the herbs. Your gardening confidence will grow with your experience.

Technical Terminology

A basic understanding of certain words is necessary if you wish to be successful. I will try to use as few technical terms as possible, to avoid confusion, but these words carry very precise meanings and their use can avoid long and cumbersome explanations.

Soil Amendment – A term used for anything you add to your soil to improve it. Examples are sand, compost, bone meal, peat moss, coconut coir. There are many more categories at garden centers and staff will be happy to explain the different possibilities and what they achieve. Unless your soil is really bad, compost will fix most problems.

Cold Spell or Cold Wave – In the United States, a cold spell is defined as the national average high temperature dropping below 20 °F (-7 °C). However, in practical usage, this refers to an unexpected drop to frost temperatures or lower.

Annual – A plant that completes its life cycle in one growing season. It germinates from seed, grows, flowers, ripens seed and then dies. Its life can be extended a bit by cutting off flowers to temporarily prevent seed formation. However, hormones stimulated by seed formation will cause the herb to die eventually, no matter what you do. Examples of annual herbs are basil, dill, and coriander.

Biennial – A plant that takes two years to complete its life cycle. These herbs usually grow as a rosette in the first growing season, become dormant for a while (normally during a cold spell), then send up a flowering shoot or spike the second summer. A few biennials you may know of are sage, parsley, and stevia.

Perennial – Lives for three or more seasons, even after ripening seed. There are short-lived perennials that die after three to five years, and you need to know this so that you won't be surprised when they die. It's nothing you did. Then there are long-lived perennials, like comfrey and trees. Some of these will live hundreds of years so plant them where you want them to remain! Commonly known perennial herbs are oregano, thyme, and chives.

Hardy – This refers to plants that survive conditions that are not conducive to growing for most plants; these are usually cold, but

also hot, dry conditions. Some plants will withstand bad conditions only for a short time, while others can handle prolonged cold spells.

Half-hardy – This term refers to a plant that can withstand light frost but hard freezes will kill it. Pot marigolds (*Calendula officinalis*) are half-hardy annuals; mature plants withstand light frosts and keep on blooming until a hard freeze finishes them off. Rosemary (*Salvia rosmarinus*) is a half-hardy perennial shrub. It survives temperatures down to 20°F (-7°C) but any lower and it will die.

Tender – These plants die at the slightest cold spell. Sweet Basil (*Ocimum basilicum*) will blacken and die at the first frost as well as when it ripens seed, so we call it a tender annual. Pineapple sage (*Salvia elegans*) is a tender perennial. It will survive indefinitely if grown where winters are warm, or brought inside in cold winter areas, but will die to the ground at a frost and die completely if temperatures stay below freezing for more than a few nights.

Wet tolerant – This term refers to herbs that prefer soggy, wet soils. Most plants need well-drained soil but some actually thrive in wet soil, laughing at seasonal flooding or growing in damp places or swamps without suffering from root rot.

Hardening off – This means to get a plant used to the outside world. Much like tanning your skin so you won't get a sunburn on vacation, hardening off allows the plant time to build up chlorophyll in its leaves and strengthen up against the wind. The plant is taken outside and placed in a protected location for two hours, then brought back inside. The next day that's repeated. On the third day, the herb stays out for four hours. The fourth day is a repeat of the third, and so on. If any plants show signs of stress, they are held at the previous day's exposure level. Every second day, the duration of the plant's exposure to outside conditions is increased until, after seven to ten days, the plant is ready to be transplanted and grown permanently outside in the ground or in a pot.

Soil pH – This is a scale that measures the acidity or alkalinity of garden soil. At certain pH levels things in the soil can become toxic or bound up and unavailable. **Acidic** soil has a pH of less than 5.5. Aluminum and manganese become more available below this pH. But nitrogen, calcium, potassium and other elements become unavailable. Lime can sweeten your soil but too much is damaging. The local agricultural center in your area can do a soil test. **Neutral** is a pH of 7. Neutral soils are 6.5 to 7.5. Soils with a pH of 7.5 and higher are called sweet, basic or **Alkaline**. Other elements become unavailable to plants when the pH is high.

One summer, when I was still mostly a beginner, I was growing herbs in rows in the traditional manner. My soil is naturally acidic, so I added limestone gravel around the coltsfoot, as it is commonly found growing along railroad tracks here. The rosemary plants growing in the next row shot up three to four feet in just a few months! I have since learned that rosemary prefers soil on the sweet side.

Stratification – This is a fancy word for the up and down cold temperatures needed by some herbs to trigger germination; it often involves freezing. The minimum length of time your seeds need to be stratified will be different for each species and falls somewhere between a few weeks and 90 days. This can be achieved by sowing seeds in the winter or by placing them in your refrigerator.

Botanical Name – Common names of plants may be different in different countries, even between different areas within a country. The botanical name is unique to each plant species and does not change, no matter what country you are in, or what language the common names are in. Many herbs have a long-standing relationship with humans, during which different varieties have been chosen for certain qualities. Factors such as color of the flower, shorter vegetative growth, hardiness, flavor or scent, and intensity of medicinal constituents, have all been altered by humans. Each plant species is classified according to how similar it is to other species. At the family level, all members share similar characteristics. Most plants in the mint family, for example, have square stems. Botanists use these similarities to try and identify unknown species of plants. At the level of a plant's genus and species, however, it is unique, and only shares its characteristics with other individuals of the same species. These two identifiers (the genus and species names) are used to give us the plant's botanical (or scientific) name.

It is important to know a plant's botanical name, or at least to know where to look for it, as this is the only way to know exactly what you're buying or growing. For example, the common name mint is applied to many very different plants. Do you want peppermint (*Mentha piperita*), spearmint (*Mentha spicata*) or maybe the curly-leaf variety of spearmint (*Mentha spicata* var. "Kentucky Colonel") preferred as a garnish for mint juleps? Or perhaps you want to grow one of the many other mints, such as chocolate mint, that is a crazy yummy type of mint. The botanical name will let you know one from another in any country, so that you buy the correct herb, seed or baby plant the first time.

The discussions of herbs in our book start with the most often used common name, then the family that it belongs to and its botanical name, which is global, so you will start seeing the similarities as well as the differences in each family.

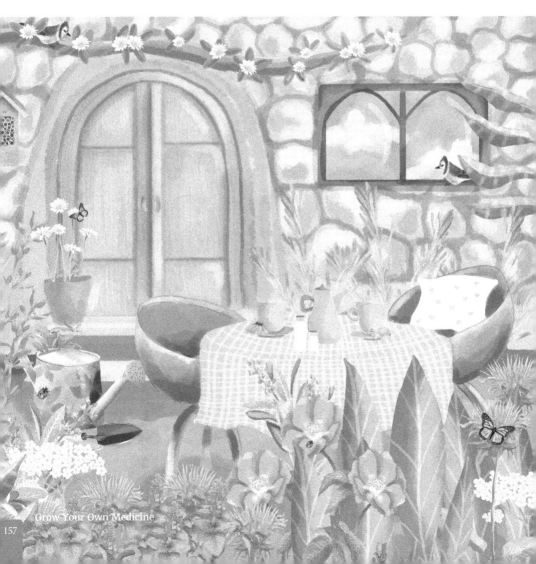

Your Unmistakably Unique Garden

When you think of starting an herb garden, you may feel a little overwhelmed because there is so much to learn. Many things are in your control, but not everything. You can't control the rain, sun, or the cold outside. It empowers you to know what is normal where you live. We are going to walk this journey together, and I want you not to worry in the least because I will teach you all the tricks that I have been taught. Before you know it, it will all be second nature to you, just like it is for me.

The secret to a successful herb garden is not about 'having a green thumb', but rather it's about how you treat your plants; it's knowing the personality of the soil, and it's feeling your way into connecting with your garden naturally. It also means having respect for it by keeping it tidy and free from weeds and harmful pests, just as you would care for your home, pets, or even children. Being a responsible gardener also means that you are water conscious. When you have all this in place, remember that not all herbs will grow easily in all areas. As we have grown in our knowledge of herbs, we began to map areas across the earth into hardiness zones. These zones make it much easier for the gardener to understand which plants will thrive outside and which ones will not. Depending on the zone that you live in, you will have more luck with some plants and find others extremely difficult or nearly impossible to grow. This is why I have mentioned the hardiness zones for all the herbs in this book, so that your gardening experience can be easier than ever. Let us learn a little more about the hardiness zones.

Hardiness Zones

Understanding which hardiness zone you live in is very important. The hardiness zone is not necessarily a limiting factor though and you must never look at it that way. By knowing what conditions your garden naturally has, you can also compensate in order for other plants to thrive. In other words, let's say that you live in Raleigh, North Carolina, in the United States. Your hardiness zone will be overlapping between 7b and 8a. This means that you already know, from looking at your hardiness zone, that you will have mild winters and low temperatures that range between

10°F (-12°C) and 20°F (-7°C). Your summers will have cooler nights with temperate climates throughout the day, allowing a longer growing season. After researching, you will realize that thyme, hibiscus, and hawthorn, among many other plants, will thrive naturally. You would begin your garden with these naturally thriving species first. Once you have mastered growing the plants that are naturally suited to your hardiness zone, you could then move on to plants that are typically found one zone above and one zone below, and so on. Sounds doable, right? That's because it really is.

If you live where the weather is extreme, you may have no choice but to grow the herb you want inside. I have a bay tree (*Laurus nobilis*) that prefers the mild winters of its native Mediterranean area (hardiness zone 9–10) which is definitely not mine. When the forecast threatens frost, I move it inside for the winter season. I also know from my research that this tree prefers light from the top instead of from the side. Knowing the bay's preferences is important, including its temperature limitations. Bay is hardy to 0°F (-18°C), but only for short periods of a few hours. Overall, it is best kept above 20°F (-7°C) . This has allowed me to grow it in a big pot in front of a picture window every winter for the last 15+ years. As Bush, Obama and Trump have come and gone, my bay tree is still growing strong.

My warm season is also short, so I start many herb plants early inside my home or in a greenhouse to transplant out later. These include species that need a long growing season to reach maturity or to get an early jump on summer.

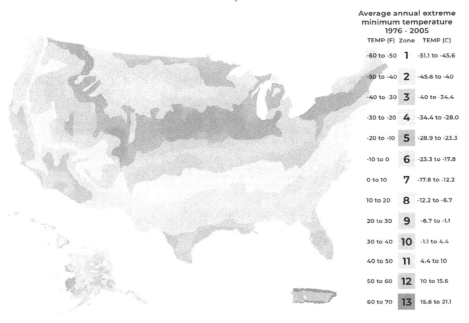

Average annual extreme
minimum temperature
1976 - 2005

TEMP (F)	Zone	TEMP (C)
-60 to -50	1	-51.1 to -45.6
-50 to -40	2	-45.6 to -40
-40 to -30	3	-40 to -34.4
-30 to -20	4	-34.4 to -28.0
-20 to -10	5	-28.9 to -23.3
-10 to 0	6	-23.3 to -17.8
0 to 10	7	-17.8 to -12.2
10 to 20	8	-12.2 to -6.7
20 to 30	9	-6.7 to -1.1
30 to 40	10	-1.1 to 4.4
40 to 50	11	4.4 to 10
50 to 60	12	10 to 15.6
60 to 70	13	15.6 to 21.1

Hardiness Zones of the United States of America

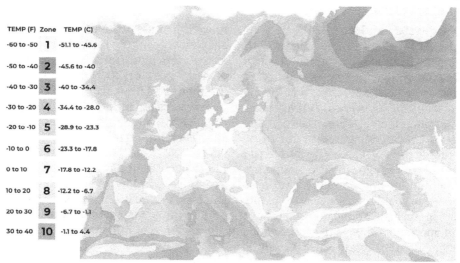

TEMP (F)	Zone	TEMP (C)
-60 to -50	1	-51.1 to -45.6
-50 to -40	2	-45.6 to -40
-40 to -30	3	-40 to -34.4
-30 to -20	4	-34.4 to -28.0
-20 to -10	5	-28.9 to -23.3
-10 to 0	6	-23.3 to -17.8
0 to 10	7	-17.8 to -12.2
10 to 20	8	-12.2 to -6.7
20 to 30	9	-6.7 to -1.1
30 to 40	10	-1.1 to 4.4

Hardiness Zones of Europe

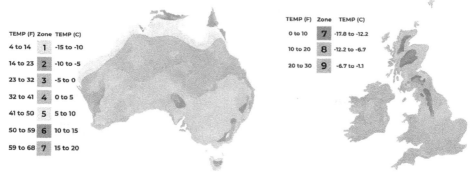

Hardiness Zones of Australia

TEMP (F)	Zone	TEMP (C)
4 to 14	1	-15 to -10
14 to 23	2	-10 to -5
23 to 32	3	-5 to 0
32 to 41	4	0 to 5
41 to 50	5	5 to 10
50 to 59	6	10 to 15
59 to 68	7	15 to 20

Hardiness Zones of Australia

TEMP (F)	Zone	TEMP (C)
0 to 10	7	-17.8 to -12.2
10 to 20	8	-12.2 to -6.7
20 to 30	9	-6.7 to -1.1

Hardiness Zones of the United Kingdom

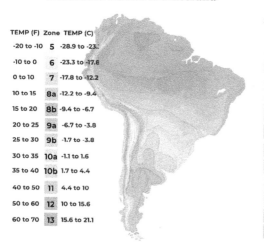

TEMP (F)	Zone	TEMP (C)
-20 to -10	5	-28.9 to -23.:
-10 to 0	6	-23.3 to -17.8
0 to 10	7	-17.8 to -12.2
10 to 15	8a	-12.2 to -9.4
15 to 20	8b	-9.4 to -6.7
20 to 25	9a	-6.7 to -3.8
25 to 30	9b	-1.7 to -3.8
30 to 35	10a	-1.1 to 1.6
35 to 40	10b	1.7 to 4.4
40 to 50	11	4.4 to 10
50 to 60	12	10 to 15.6
60 to 70	13	15.6 to 21.1

Hardiness Zones of South America

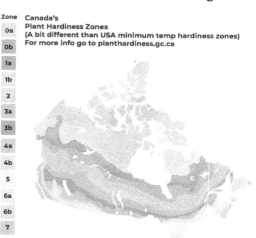

Zone	Canada's
0a	**Plant Hardiness Zones**
0b	(A bit different than USA minimum temp hardiness zones)
1a	For more info go to planthardiness.gc.ca
1b	
2	
3a	
3b	
4a	
4b	
5	
6a	
6b	
7	

Hardiness Zones of Canada

Climate

Seasonal climate changes are the main factors used when classifying a hardiness zone. So, the information pertaining to a hardiness zone will indicate the lowest annual temperature averaged over a certain number of years. The coldest temperatures occur in the hardiness zones with the lowest numbers (Zone 1 and 2), while zones with higher numbers experience warmer average annual temperatures. The higher numbers may also indicate zones that are prone to having a period of drought that divides the growing season. When I first moved to Tennessee I thought I'd have a six-month growing season. Instead, I got two short seasons – one before the hot drought and one after. Even the trees sometimes lose their leaves during the dry spell, creating a second spring when it begins to rain again. I also learned to grow around these hot dry times by increasing how often I water and even providing shade when possible. I especially do this with my container plants on my porch, by using a canopy. It really works too! I am able to have a large variety of flowers, herbs, and even veggies all summer long.

Each of the hardiness zones is separated from the next by a difference of ten degrees in lowest annual average temperature. Some areas may contain several different hardiness zones. This is normal and it is important to remember that these are simply climate averages that may be changing.

Some herbs hate dry, hot air, while others don't tolerate high humidity. This also may be part of your climate.

If you are not yet very experienced in caring for plants which would thrive in different climate conditions, then sticking to your hardiness zone's native herbs is best until you feel comfortable enough to venture beyond its safety.

Humidity

Humidity is a measure of how much water vapor is found in the air. Plants mostly thrive in 50% humidity conditions. However, this is not true for all plants. Think of a tropical forest where humidity levels are really high. Plants here are adapted to the high humidity and would find it difficult, or nearly impossible, to survive in arid regions where humidity levels are 25% and lower.

All your plants 'breathe' and 'sweat'. This in and out is called respiration and transpiration. Transpiration concerns moisture. On the underside of the leaves of your plants are stomata (minute openings). The stomata close when it is too hot for the plant, and they open when temperatures have normalized. The evaporation of water through the stomata ensures your plant can draw dissolved nutrients up from the soil, but when temperatures are too hot and there is not enough water vapor in the air, this loss of water will eventually cause your plant to wilt and die.

So, how do we test to see what the humidity of the air is? The easiest method is by using a hygrometer. You are more likely to find a decent thermometer and hygrometer together. They're inexpensive and a great addition to your inside and outside garden. If you do not want to purchase a hygrometer, looking at the weather forecast gives a rough idea, although this will often be the average humidity over a large area. The third method only works indoors and it involves a glass of ice cubes. Place three ice cubes in a glass. Leave for ten to fifteen minutes. When you return, you should find water vapor on the sides of the glass. If there is no sign of any water droplets, then your house is too dry and your plants will suffer as a result.

One way to increase the humidity is to fill a saucer with stones and place your pot on top, keeping the saucer full of water just to the top of the stones. The water will evaporate and add humidity to the immediate vicinity of the plant. If you are growing more than a few plants, a humidifier is a great addition for both your plants and for you. If your home is prone to low humidity, your plants may suffer more pests and you may suffer dry mucous membranes and skin.

I used to live in Arizona before and, let me tell you, it was as dry as the Sahara! I used to get dry skin and my hubby had severe asthmatic problems all the time. We invested in a humidifier and it really helped us, as well as our plants. Dry air is not healthy, not for us humans, and not for our plants. Desert plants have adapted to this dryness, others have not. Take tarragon, for example. No matter how often you water it, it will wither away when the air is hot and dry. It grows best where temperatures are moderate ... like England's weather ...

Designing Your Garden

Start by making a list of the herbs you want to grow and use, and research each plant's growing needs. Needs include type of soil, amount of water, space and, where appearance counts, color of foliage and blooms. You may need to plant in more than one place in order to meet those needs. Do your herbs prefer full sun or partial shade? Do you live where a little protection would be appreciated? Does the soil meet the herb's needs or does it need to be amended? Is your list practical, or can it be shortened to start with? I always plant at least one row more than I can weed. If I ever win the lottery, I will hire a gardener whose primary job is to weed between my plants! When your list is practical, move on.

The traditional garden of long rows was convenient when using machines to do the work and for monocropping large fields. It is still used, but is not the best way to grow herbs in your backyard. Most backyards don't have large fields anymore. Your grow space may be limited to pots outside or even on a balcony.

Many herbs are grown in small patches which contain mixtures of annuals and perennials; this doesn't work well with machines. Lastly, the wide variety of herbs have different needs for light and water and so should be grown with other plants that have similar needs. I have a garden bed that gets full sun, one that gets at least partial shade, and even one that's fully shaded. How much you plant will also depend on your plans for your herbs, whether they will be for culinary, medicinal, or decorative use.

Outdoor Gardening Methods

Then, before you begin buying or

planting new plants, it is important to draw a map. This is an extremely important step and will make sure that you do not forget anything. On your map, draw the boundary area for where you want your garden to be. Work out where the sun will be the strongest in summer and in winter. Find out which areas will have more shade. Mark these areas out on your map. I did not do this in my first year of gardening. I absolutely regretted it because I should have planted some things where I had, instead, planted others. It created more work and I believe also caused my plants not to grow to their full potential.

Take a few minutes to look at your area's hardiness zone and see which species will do well, and which of those you would like to plant. If you want to concentrate on a medicinal garden then keep in mind which herbs will help your family. Likewise if you'd rather have a culinary herb garden. Remember though that many plants are dual purpose, such as mint, oregano, thyme, rosemary, and even lavender. These are my favorite types of herbs to grow because of their many uses.

As you draw your map, remember each of the plants and how they grow. Wormwood can grow happily in a pot outside, but when planted in a garden, know that it will spread both by seed and by underground roots. The same goes for mugwort, although this herb is far easier to contain and is not as happy in a pot. Thyme will also spread, once established, but it will not take over your garden. Mint is well known for taking over gardens quickly, so most people prefer to plant it in pots. Understanding how your plants will grow together is vital in achieving

success with your outdoor garden.

Another excellent addition that I swear by is the use of cover crops in vacant beds. Not only do my cover crops shade my soil but they prevent soil erosion and increase the soil fertility. Cover crops are also great for smothering weeds. I don't know anyone in my family who enjoys weeding. Some weeds are actually useful, but if you do not keep them under your thumb they will suffocate your garden. I discovered this the hard way when I lost control of them in my earliest garden. So, when you don't like something, find a good way around it. In this case we use mulch and cover crops. One excellent cover crop that seeds well is fenugreek. I love fenugreek because it does the heavy lifting for me, it breaks up my soil, adds the nitrogen needed, keeps perennial weeds and pests away and has medicinal properties. Since it's an annual it doesn't hang around. I couldn't ask for a greater gardening buddy. No wonder the Romans, Persians, Egyptians and Greeks loved this plant so much!

Traditional Gardens & Terracing

Traditional gardening by tilling a whole garden bed and then planting in rows will work with annuals but is not compatible with biennials or perennials.

My grandmother did not have the luxury of raised beds, but she did know a lot about terracing. She lived for many years in a beautiful, cozy, country house with a steep hill at the back. She had dug into that ground and had turned it into the most exquisite set of garden steps you have ever seen. It helped with the heavy downpours of rain, and assisted the plants in keeping most of the rainwater instead of losing it down

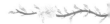

the hill, where it would have made a swamp outside her home. Terracing and raised beds are excellent additions to your garden. They require hard work and your time, but when you're done, I promise you, you won't look back. These options are investments in a community garden there are some questions you need answered. How big is the plot? How much does it cost? Do you have to pay everything upfront or can you pay rent monthly? Do you have to buy all the necessary tools? Some places provide nothing,

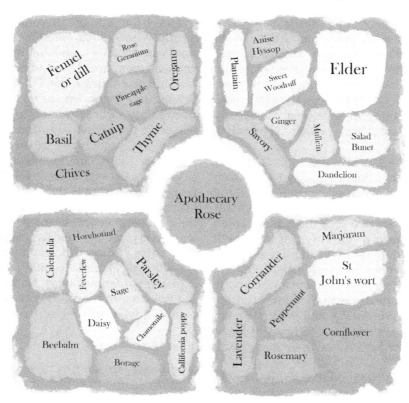

into the future of your garden. others have a communal hose, and a few provide all the basics.

Community Gardens

This type of gardening allows apartment dwellers and renters, whose landlords often won't allow the lawn to be tilled, to garden. They are also often found on college campuses for use by the students.

Before you commit to renting a space

What are you permitted to grow? Many places don't allow perennials as they aren't compatible with machine tilling of the area. Even places with raised beds may require everything to be removed by a certain date. That will limit what you can grow. Annuals and some perennially grown annuals such as dill, basil, thyme, sage and calendula, will still be worth growing. Your garden doesn't have to be either or. Annual herbs can be grown alongside vegetables and this can actually improve the growth of both. This practice is referred to as companion gardening. It is a wonderful thing to learn about, no matter where you live.

What is the removal date? Is there a specific place to leave produce that is available to share, or do you have to transport extra to your local food bank? The community garden provides space for those who wouldn't otherwise have a garden; it is truly wonderful.

Raised beds

Raised beds drain well and are best used in areas where it rains often. They also allow you to choose the soil and additives, such as compost, to fill the beds, which is a real bonus when native soil is rocky or consists of subsoil from construction. Even if you do choose to improve other areas of soil, your raised beds will allow you to start your garden straight away. There is much to be said for immediate gratification!

When I first learned about raised beds, I asked myself, "Why would I want to do this? Wouldn't it mean more unnecessary work?" – but then I moved into my

house, seven years ago. My new space had the worst soil you can think of. It was rocky, hard, and mostly clay. It also tends to rain a lot at times (when we're not dealing with a drought) and, if you recall, clay soil doesn't drain well at all. I remember standing outside, my hands on my hips, my big straw hat on my head, listening to my grandmother's soft voice in my head. She said, "When a problem seems too big, cut it down into bite-sized chunks." This is what I did. My husband built raised beds of various sizes for me, and I filled them with my idea of perfect soil to the depth I preferred. As a bonus, weeds were easier to keep under control because they didn't have their deep roots already established. For a while, I planted in the raised beds and today my outside soil is better. I still use my raised beds and I have now successfully grown the most incredible plants in the outside soil, which would never have been possible before I had the chance to condition the natural soil over time. Raised beds can be pricey, unless you have a friend who has old timber lying around. They don't have to be, though. I actually have two herb gardens I put together this past summer from broken grills. I've also made them from kiddie pools. You just need some creativity if finances are an issue. If you have the capital and/or the imagination, and you feel a raised bed would be better, do it. You won't be sorry. I sure wasn't.

Another plus is that if you build them so that you can reach the whole bed from either side, you can avoid compacting soil with foot traffic and machines. My beds are twice my arm's reach. Raised beds can also be built high enough to accommodate the disabled. This

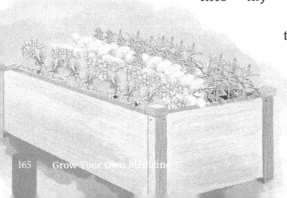

garden is yours; adjust it to your needs.

Sunken gardens

You may live where the weather is very dry. Sunken beds are basically the opposite of raised beds. Beds are dug so that the top, the growing area, is several inches below the soil around it. This allows the beds to collect every drop of water that falls there, be it from rain or from your hose. It also protects plants a bit from the hot wind because this passes right over the growing space. Sunken beds often allow you to grow herbs that would otherwise wither up and die.

Growing in a Container

When planting in containers, you need to understand the different plant containers and what works for you. Container gardening works indoors and out. You may choose to garden in pots outside, in order to control herbs that might become invasive, such as the mint varieties I mentioned earlier. The containers may be above ground to be more portable, or buried with only two inches sticking out to stop those runners. Either way, the pots need drain holes or all but swamp herbs will suffer root rot, which can be fatal for a plant.

When you decide which pot to buy, make sure that you look at the diameter of the pot's rim. The correct size is actually extremely important. For every plant, you will want to purchase a container that is just a bit bigger than the root structure. I know that this seems silly, and you would rather want a larger pot for a smaller plant to grow into, but most herbs grow roots straight down to the bottom and then around. They will fill a big pot better if

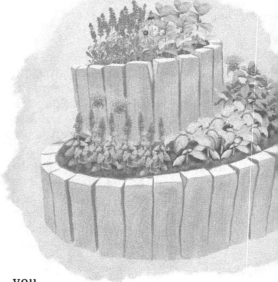

you slowly transplant up in size.

Overwatering is very easy if the pot is too big for your plant. On the other hand, if you choose a pot that is too small, you will have to water it very frequently as small pots dry out fast when they are full of roots but contain little soil to hold the water. The herb needs to be repotted if you need to water more than every other day. Your soil mixture also has a lot to do with this. Repotting will happen more often when you work like this, but you would rather want a healthy plant, than one that dies from rotting roots.

Wooden Containers

Wooden containers can be quite decorative. That's why I have two by my front door, planted with several useful and attractive herbs. Thyme hangs over the front of both. Lavender, lemon balm and marjoram grow behind in one, and pot marigolds, lemon grass, and holy basil grow in the other. I only have to step out of my door for morning tea.

Avoid treated wood. The chemicals

that deter wood-rotting organisms can also poison your plants. Apart from the fact that you would not wish to eat anything grown in a chemically-treated container, the chemicals may also stunt or kill your herbs.

Use natural wood or use a liner. Without a liner, the wood will rot in 3–5 years, depending on the type of wood. Hardwoods last longer than pine. Cedar, redwood, and locust contain natural rot resistance. If you choose a liner be sure it has drainage holes.

Concrete, Stone and Terracotta

Concrete is also magnificent in the right setting, and concrete containers will keep the colder temperatures out. I don't like them because they are heavy and cumbersome. They are great if they are going to stay in one place, though. I would also not make concrete my first choice if I needed something sturdy, but would rather opt for stone. Concrete is very alkaline and that may harm your herbs.

Most stone pots are big. Big pots keep out the frost and protect the plants. They also have a tendency to grow beautiful mosses on them and look better as they age.

Terracotta pots are a popular and commonly seen choice but can leach water quickly, which means that the soil inside soon requires more watering. These tend to be better for herbs that prefer drier soils, such as rosemary or lavender.

Grow Bags

These are great for use by renters in properties where gardens may be temporary. They can also buy you time to improve the surrounding soil when you don't want to wait to garden. Maybe your soil is rocky or needs more amending than you can do in one spring. Grow bags are much cheaper than raised beds unless all the material for your beds is found or made of recycled substances. You can also just cut a hole or holes in a large bag of potting soil and plant your herbs inside. This will only last one summer as the sun degrades the plastic, but it works. Fabric grow bags last longer. Plants potted in grow bags will grow crooked roots, which is not good if you want to harvest the roots. I have found that herbs grown in grow bags need watering as often as those grown in pots of a comparable size.

Garden Towers

Garden towers can be quite beautiful. They make great dividers, to hide something, or to put on an existing fence. While not appropriate for all plants, they can produce a big harvest from a small area. Many culinary herbs such as thyme, basil, and chives grow fine in a tower as do medicinal herbs grown for leaves or aerial parts.

Indoor Gardening Methods

Indoor gardening has its pros and its cons. I do both indoor and outdoor gardening and my entire house is filled with seedlings and fully fledged plants, including plant rescues that are brought to me. I have special dedicated places in my house where I can control the heat, the light, the water, and the humidity. And, of course, there are no pests. This does not mean pests do not come into my home. Sometimes an infected plant will make it to my doorstep and for this I have a special room, away from my other plants, where the lighting is specific and I can really heal and rescue the plant. This is referred to as a quarantine and is an important step to ensure that pests and diseases do not spread.

When gardening indoors, you will either choose to grow plants inside your house or to build a greenhouse in which to grow your herbs. A greenhouse is a wonderful idea and it allows immense control over the plants. Our greenhouse is not big, but it houses the herbs I want to protect from our cold season, herbs I want access to during winter, and those early babies that need to get a head start before going into my outdoor garden. My husband tells me all the time that we are running out of space. I constantly run out of land in which to plant, but somehow I always manage to find a tiny place.

Container gardening

When planting in containers, indoors or out, you need to understand the different plant containers and what works for you. I swear by terracotta pots but that is simply because they allow the soil to 'breathe'. I also love terracotta because it can be put in the garden as is. But, as I mentioned previously, these pots can leach water from the soil faster than you may want.

Plastic Pots are cheap and affordable on any budget. These 'starter pots' are made from petroleum and often end up in a landfill, so many gardeners won't use them but recycling can relieve some of the objection to them. They're also not very pretty. I have many different sizes that originally came from purchases. Plastic pots naturally prevent evaporation from the sides, thus reducing watering needs.

One problem with plastic is that sunlight makes it brittle; better quality pots have sun protection additives and this means that better pots will last several years before degrading.

You can also buy thicker plastic pots from any store and still save a considerable amount of money. Thicker plastic pots are more durable than the starter pots that plants usually come in.

Recycled Containers are very economical and prevent your local landfill from filling up too quickly. Be sure your chosen container has enough drainage and add more holes if necessary. This is best done before disinfecting. Then wash your recycled container well. Disinfect by soaking for at least ten minutes in one part chlorine bleach to nine parts water. This mixture is used in many greenhouses. It's an affordable liquid to disinfect not only seedling flats and pots, but benches too. I don't want to spread any disease.

Unglazed Ceramic Pots dry out faster than other pots because of the porous nature of ceramics. They are useful for plants that prefer dry, well drained soils. But they have a down side. Mineral salts build up on the outside of your pot as a white film and can damage your herbs unless scrubbed off. I wash mine at the end of every summer or after transplanting.

Pots are great for allowing you to control water levels for herbs that need to dry out between waterings. Glazing or painting the interior of the pot will make it behave more like a plastic pot and slow evaporation through the sides. Painting the outside of the pot can be decorative.

My aloe, rose geranium, and other herbs that need to come inside during frost season, are in pots. I have also successfully grown veggies on my porch using containers.

Buy or collect a variety of sizes. Having pots ready when you need them will reduce your temptation to use a pot that is too big or too small. Commercial pots come in many sizes, starting with seedling flats and cell packs, and moving up to giant ones. My bay tree is currently growing in one that is 18 inches wide and fairly deep, but there are larger pots. Pots that are two feet or more in diameter are often referred to as planters.

Make sure to get extra plastic pots, particularly the starter pots, just in case you need them for a new cutting or a seedling. You will not be sorry for having extra pots on hand.

Knowing the different pot sizes, their diameters and volumes, really helps when shopping for containers online.

Pot Size	Diameter	Pot Size	Diameter
US Gallon	Inches	Liters	Cm
0.125 (pint)	4"	0.47	10.2
0.25 (quart)	5" to 6"	0.95	12.7 to 15.24
1	7" to 8"	3.8	17.8 to 20.3
2	8½" to 9"	7.6	21.6 to 22.9
3	10"	11.4	25.4
5	12"	18.9	30.5
7	14"	26.5	35.6

Must-Have Gardening Tools

There are thousands of gardening tools that you can choose to use in your garden. I have a few trusty ones that have been with me for so long that I could not bear to get rid of them. Then there are those gardening tools that are absolutely essential but that need to be replaced every so often. Gardening gloves are one of those. I have pink, turquoise, green and really old, leather ones. I have so many because I cannot

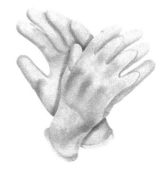

ever garden without my gloves. The soil gets under my fingernails, it stains my hands and, even though I love digging my hands into the rich soil, the cleaning up afterwards has become something that I am not so fond of. Gloves should be the first item on your list, in my opinion, and you need to have three or four pairs in the garden. Sometimes they get wet, sometimes they get completely ruined; whatever the case, I believe we can never have too many pairs. I know some people who never use gloves to garden though, so it's up to personal preference.

Your next two friends in the garden are your spade and your garden fork. The soil should always be turned and tilled, and this is the job of your garden fork. It may seem like a lot of work at first but you want to till the land that you will use to a depth of about 8–10 inches or 20-25 cm. You only need to till the land once though. When you do it too often, you're actually breaking up the soil structure and harming the web of life, underneath the ground, that is vital for a healthy garden. You do not need to till the soil in raised beds, however; since you don't walk in them, the soil won't become compacted.

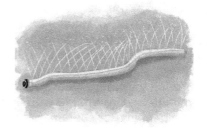

Our ancestors across the globe tilled the lands, historically. Unfortunately they did not understand the damage that this does, until very recently. So, you will till and turn your soil only when you begin your garden. If your garden is going to be fairly large, you can also use a mechanical tiller. After the initial tilling, your garden fork will be used for many other things in the garden, such as transplantation of plants, removing deep-rooted weeds and mixing compost. Your spade is your digger. You really want to get a very sturdy spade that will hold your weight when digging new holes. In addition to the spade, smaller hand trowels are wonderful for small gardening projects. It is not essential that you have more than one but it is nice to have about three different ones at your disposal.

There are a few essential elements in the garden and the most obvious is water. A durable, lengthy water hose must be high on your first gardening shopping list. Purchase a leaky hose if you can afford to. Get an adjustable nozzle if you can't. They are both wonderful for the plants but both a leaky hose and drip irrigation deliver water to the roots and avoid wetting leaves, thereby conserving water. Sprinklers shoot water into the air and increase evaporation and water loss. They also wet leaves, increasing the chance of spreading disease. Placing hoses under mulch to protect the plastic from the sun will allow them to last longer.

You will also want to get some sort of hose reel to wrap the hose on when you have finished using it. Mine sits neatly on the wall, out of sight and out of mind for my two dogs, who find eating the hose preferable to chewing bones. You could also use a hose pot. Check out the resources in the end, in our website we have the direct links to some high quality tools that we have cherry picked.

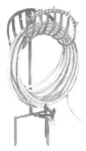

There is one more essential item without which no garden is complete – that is a wheelbarrow. We all believe we are super strong until we begin gardening. A wheelbarrow will save you time and make sure you aren't tired out before the gardening even begins. When purchasing a wheelbarrow, do yourself a favor and don't get a plastic one, or one that looks as though it couldn't handle a large stack of bricks. You want your wheelbarrow to last. Make sure to store your wheelbarrow in the garage or an outbuilding to prevent weather damage and rust. You can make, or have made, a hardware cloth sieve to assist you with removing small rocks.

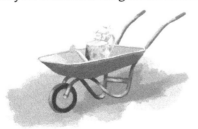

Kneeling down to plant or pull weeds can be painful. A stool or pad for your knees is nice to have and will protect your knees and keep them dry.

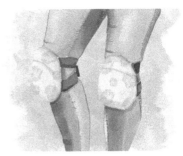

Agricultural fabric or cloches (domes) will protect plants from early frost, extend the fall growing season, provide shade where needed, and protect your plants from insect damage. Agricultural cloth is great for making tunnels to protect many plants, while cloches protect individual plants. I often make cloches from transparent milk jugs and clear, 2-liter bottles with the bottoms cut off. I remove the caps every morning to encourage circulation and replace them in the evening to retain the day's heat. Both of these devices trap the day's heat given off by the soil on cool, spring nights that dip to frost. I watch the daily weather forecast closely in spring and fall.

Flea beetles live in the soil and mulch. They caused me no end of trouble until I learned to make a tunnel to protect my basil.

Now that you are familiar with the basics, we'll move on to the specific herbs. Control your lusting, if you can. It'll likely be difficult though. I know it is for me.

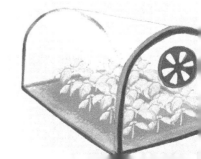

21 Lucky Medicinal Herbs to Kickstart Your Garden

Each plant listed below is named firstly by its common name, and then by the family to which it belongs. Lastly, its botanical or scientific name is given. The botanical name is usually in the form of two words ... first the genus and then the species. For example, *Salvia officinalis* is the botanical name of what is commonly called sage. *Salvia* is the genus to which the plant belongs, and *officinalis* is its species. If the plant is a specific cultivar (variety), then the name of the variety is also added to the botanical name. For example, *Salvia officinalis* var. "Berggarten." Lastly, the common name of the herb species is listed.

Symbols to indicate different uses

These symbols are made for you so you can quickly see the herb page and recognize the main uses. They are:

Medicinal

Culinary

Decorative

Tea

Dye

Scent

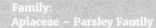
Flat-leaf Parsley

Family:
Apiaceae – Parsley Family

Botanical Name:
Petroselinum crispum variety *neapolitanum*

Other Common Names:
Italian Parsley; has many cultivars.

I tried to grow parsley from seed as a child, and it never worked. Then Nana taught me that I should grow parsley from seed only once the soil is warm; this is because parsley hates being transplanted. To get a jump on summer, in short season areas, start parsley transplants in peat pots or soil blocks. You want to plant the whole thing without disturbing the roots, as breaking the tap root most often results in a stunted plant.

Native to the eastern and central Mediterranean area, parsley is now grown worldwide. Flat-leaf parsley is the closest to its wild cousins. It is a little easier to grow than the curly-leaf variety and grows outside in zones 3–9. Parsley grows best in full sun and moist, well-drained soil and, while tolerant of rain, dislikes soggy soil. Parsley can handle shade when grown in hotter climates, especially during the sunniest hours (10am–2pm). Since parsley is a biennial, it flowers early in the 2nd growing season, BUT, if you want to delay it from seeding, you should cut its flower stalks while they are still budded.

Parsley is tolerant of indoor growing as long as light is bright. Parsley is a common indoor and greenhouse crop. It also does well as an outdoor container plant and in wall gardens.

Propagation

Propagation is by seed and many lawn and garden centers sell seedlings in the spring. Germination for the seed is notoriously slow. Parsley can take four to six weeks to germinate because of chemical compounds called furanocoumarins in the seed coat. Mothers often taught their daughters that the seed had to go down to visit the devil seven times before it could sprout. As mentioned before, you should plant seed directly into its permanent home, or don't break the tap root when transplanting. Thin out seedlings (remove all but the healthiest seedlings) to be about ten inches apart.

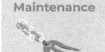

Feed parsley with a bi-monthly top dressing of compost. If you are working with a first year garden and your soil is not so great, use ½ strength fish emulsion or organic fertilizer. Parsley is a heavy feeder and will need to replace all those leaves you'll be harvesting. In the fall, if you're going to grow it as an annual, remove the plants and ready the area for next spring. If you intend to winter the herb over (which I recommend), wait until next spring to remove any dead leaves once signs of new growth are visible.

Indoor care is as easy as outdoor care. Water when your finger tells you the soil is dry. Empty the saucer under each pot after every watering so the roots won't sit in water. Feed half-strength fish emulsion or half-strength compost water monthly, as the roots have limited soil.

Common Problems

My first year growing parsley brought an unexpected surprise. I found swallowtail butterfly caterpillars on them and was dismayed when the insects ate many leaves. I quickly learned to plant enough parsley plants for them and me. I did this instead of just getting rid of them because they are important pollinators. Outside there are few diseases that are a problem but you must make sure the soil is well drained so that the plants do not get root or crown rot, especially when unusual wet seasons hit. We also have rabbits, groundhogs and other pests in our lush garden that love to make my plants their own personal buffet. Inside, though, it's a different story. Be careful with blight disease inside your greenhouse. It gets carried on seeds. There are cultivars that are blight resistant. Indoors or out, thin out the seedlings to encourage good air circulation. Healthy plants, air circulation and sunlight prevent most diseases.

Medicinal Use

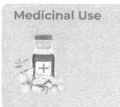

Parsley is low in calories and contains many vitamins, especially vitamins A, C , and K (which controls blood clotting and bone health), and minerals. It is used as an antioxidant to prevent cellular damage from free radicals. It's also a diuretic, making it valuable in the fight against urinary tract infections, kidney stones, and water retention. It also plays a part in treating diabetes, asthma, and high blood pressure, and in starting menstrual flow. A friend of mine didn't have a menstrual cycle for three months. She was worried and came to me because she knows how I am with my herbs. I told her that parsley could help her out. She was skeptical but it worked for her. Parsley is used to keep your body healthy and prevent many serious conditions, including heart disease, eye issues, and even cancers.

Safety

Parsley is regarded as safe when used as a flavoring and in normal culinary amounts. It is safe for most internal uses, in medicinal amounts, for a short time. A short time, for most, is three months or less. In some users, parsley can cause an allergic skin rash. Do not use medicinal amounts if pregnant. Long-term use of large amounts can cause anemia or irritate your kidneys. Parsley seed oil makes your skin extra sensitive and it will burn easily when exposed to the sun.

Culinary use

Flat-leaf parsley's flavor is stronger than that of the curly-leaf variety, and it stands up to long cooking times, including in Italian dishes (a personal favorite of my family's) such as marinara sauce and lasagna, as well as soups, stews, potato dishes, meats, and other casseroles. It is so popular that there are many cultivars, including the Radiicosum group (aka Hamburg parsley), with flat leaves but bred for its big root that is eaten as a vegetable.

Harvest

Leaves destined for cooking may be harvested anytime that they are large enough. Harvest for medicine when the flavor and scent are strongest, after at least 70–90 days of growth. Harvest seeds when close to ripe but before they shatter. Roots are dug up when big enough, which is usually in the fall of the first growing season.

One delicious and interesting use for parsley is to put it in what English speakers call 'soup bags.' The French call them *bouquet garni* but both names refer to a mixture of herbs that is commonly used to flavor a soup or broth pot, meats and casseroles. Although there is a wide variety of herbs that can be added, parsley, thyme and bay leaves are always used as a base. Fresh herbs are often used but dried herbs may be used as well. Bags of dried herbs are convenient as they can be made up ahead of time and stored until needed.

Soup Bag for a Chicken (or Veggie) Broth

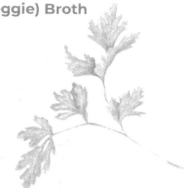

To make one soup bag:
1 bay leaf
1 sprig of sage
2 sprigs of thyme
2 sprigs of marjoram
½ of a stalk of leafy celery
4 sprigs flat-leaf parsley
3–4 black peppercorns, whole

- Tie all herbs in a cheesecloth square or small bag and add to the stock pot.

- Remove before serving the food.

- If making ahead, use dried herbs and convert sprigs to teaspoons and use 1/3 the amount.

- Store dried herb soup bags, until needed, in a tightly sealed jar in a cool dark place.

- Use rosemary for beef, instead of sage, for fish substitute the sage and marjoram with tarragon.

Curly-leaf Parsley

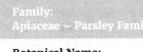

Family:
Apiaceae – Parsley Family

Botanical Name:
Petroselinum crispum var. *crispum*

Common name:
Curled-leaf Parsley, Garden Parsley

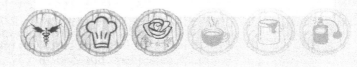

Ancient Greeks considered parsley the symbol of death. They spread it over graves and made funeral wreaths with it. It was also spread around a dead body to control the odor. British folklore held that parsley only grew well in a household where the woman wore the pants.

Curly-leaf parsley is a little harder to grow than the flat-leaf variety, although most of what's true for flat-leaf parsley is also true for this variety. Curly-leaf parsley is a bit milder and very attractive looking, and is my preferred choice for fresh and decorative use. I use it in green and macaroni salads and it is a basic ingredient in tabouli (aka tabbouleh). Everyone is familiar with curly-leaf parsley as a garnish, but what is lesser known is that the parsley garnish is meant to be chewed after the rest of the meal is finished, because it will sweeten your breath. Nana taught me that the high chlorophyll content clears your breath of the aromas of onions and garlic, to make it smell sweet.

Both parsleys grow best in moist, well-drained soil, with full sun. Both grow best between 72 and 86°F (20–30°C), but tolerate a wide range of temperatures. Mature plants are cold tolerant and, although they won't grow in the snow, you can brush it aside to harvest parsley that grew earlier in the season. Curly-leaf parsley is a biennial, flowering early in the second growing season. Cutting off the flower while in bud will delay blooming, but the leaves will develop a bit of bitterness once flower stalks form.

Typically, plants grown for the leaf crop are spaced 4 –6 inches apart, while those grown as a root crop are spaced 8 inches apart to allow room for the root development.

Propagation, Maintenance, Pests and diseases, Medicinal Use and safety precautions are the same as for flat-leaf parsley.

Culinary use

Curly-leaf parsley is milder than the flat-leaf variety. For fresh use, it is the parsley of my choice. Parsley makes a plate beautiful when used as a garnish. Added to many green salads, parsley is the main ingredient in tabouli and vegetable casseroles.

Other Uses

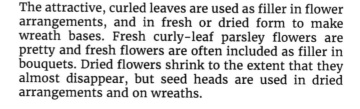

The attractive, curled leaves are used as filler in flower arrangements, and in fresh or dried form to make wreath bases. Fresh curly-leaf parsley flowers are pretty and fresh flowers are often included as filler in bouquets. Dried flowers shrink to the extent that they almost disappear, but seed heads are used in dried arrangements and on wreaths.

Harvest

Harvest I harvest the aerial parts, seed, and roots for medicinal use and outside leaves for culinary use as soon as they are large enough. The inner leaves of the rosette will continue to grow, providing future harvests. Leaves grown for medicinal use may be harvested when needed but are strongest just before blooming, late in the first growing season or early in the second. Seeds are harvested when ripe but before they shatter. Harvest roots in the first autumn.

Simple Tabouli Recipe

½ cup bulgur wheat

½ cup boiling water

1 cup cucumber, diced

1 cup tomato, diced or cherry tomatoes, halved

1 teaspoon salt

3 bunches curly-leaf parsley, fresh and diced

⅓ cup spearmint leaves, fresh and chopped finely

⅓ cup green onion, including green parts, sliced thinly

1 garlic clove

⅓ cup EVOO (extra virgin olive oil)

4 tablespoons lemon juice, or to taste

- Mix ½ teaspoon salt with diced tomato and cucumber and let rest for ten minutes. Pour off excess juice. Rinse off excess salt.

- Combine bulgar wheat with boiling water. Let stand until cool. All the water will be absorbed.

- Mix all ingredients together.

- Let stand at least 15 minutes to allow all flavors to combine.

- Serve tabouli at room temperature or chilled. Will keep 3–4 days, refrigerated.

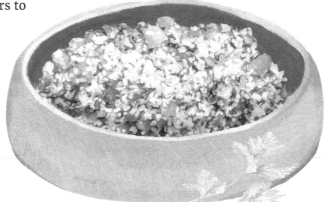

Yarrow

Family:
Asteraceae – Daisy family

Botanical Name:
Achillea millefolium

Other Common Names:
Milfoil, Thousand-leaf, Soldier's Woundwort,
Sanguinary, Yarroway

Achillea millefolium is a perennial native to North America. It has finely cut, even, fern-like leaves. It grows flower stalks that are four times the height of those leaves, often to 36 inches (91 cm) when blooming. It blooms from early- to mid-summer (the end of May to July in the Northern Hemisphere) and has white, flat-topped umbels of flowers. Yarrow prefers well-drained soil in full sun, but will tolerate some shade and less than optimal soils. It is not particular about pH and hardy in zones 3–9.

There are other species hybrids with flowers in shades of yellow, red, or pink. Nearly every garden center or flower catalog carries at least one. The plant is very drought tolerant and has flowers that attract pollinators and butterflies.

Propagation

Seeds need light to germinate and will sprout in two to three weeks. This herb grows in clumps that slowly widen and can be divided, or you can purchase a transplant. I always plant, or transplant, seedlings 24 inches apart.

Maintenance

All yarrows are low maintenance herbs. When grown in a container, I only water them when the soil is dry at a depth of two knuckles. In the garden, they only need watering during a long drought. I add a bit of compost in the spring; that's the only fertilizer they need. The plants do get leggy if too much nitrogen is available. Deadhead them if you don't harvest. Divide clumps every four or five years.

Yarrows don't usually have problems when I grow them. Herbs planted in shady areas sometimes experience spittle bugs or aphids. Yarrow can develop powdery mildew or botrytis in humid seasons. Low growing, fuzzy varieties suffer rot if not kept well drained.

Medicinal Use

Common yarrow is astringent, antimicrobial, and analgesic. The dried and powdered leaves are used to stop bleeding. I have it in my first aid kit when hubby and I go on hikes. A cooled infusion is used to treat earaches, as a wash for cuts, scrapes, and minor wounds to prevent or treat infection and as a gargle for feverish colds, sore throats, mouth or gum sores and tooth issues. It has flavonoids and alkaloids that improve digestion, relieve loss of appetite, as well as other gastrointestinal issues. Those same flavonoids and alkaloids can help relieve depression and anxiety.

Safety

Rarely, yarrow can cause an allergic rash. Long-term use, including use of the essential oil, can make your skin more sensitive to the sun. Cover up and apply sunscreen if using this herb long-term. Long-term use may also cause sperm abnormalities. Yarrow should be used only under professional supervision if you are dealing with kidney disease.

Yarrow is toxic to cats, dogs, and horses. Symptoms of yarrow poisoning are vomiting, diarrhea, increased urination and dermatitis.

Culinary use

Common yarrow has a bitter yet delicate, grass-like flavor. Before the discovery of the brewing properties of hops, yarrow was often used in the making of beer. The revival of the craft beer industry has increased its use. Yarrow is included in some bitters, liquors, and tea blends (a common means of ingestion for medicinal use). Chopped leaves are added to salads, eggs, soups, and casseroles..

Other Uses

All yarrow flowers (and long flower stems) dry well for use in wreaths, swags and other dried floral and herbal arrangements. Yarrow is used to prevent erosion, due to its deep roots and drought resistance, and is sometimes grown as a non-grass lawn that tolerates mowing as long as it's not cut too short. Before the invention of plastic, pick-up sticks (a game) were made from yarrow stems, which grow very straight and dry hard. All species of this herb are used in companion planting to attract predatory wasps, lady bugs, and other beneficial insects. And it WORKS! Yarrow can be used to make a long-lasting dye for greens and yellows, depending on mordant and fabric used.

Harvest

Leaves are strongest just before, or when, a few flowers are open. I harvest flowers when half the umbel flowers are open.

Chamomile

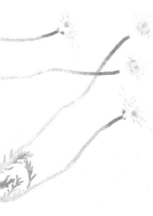

Botanical Name:
Matricaria chamomilla

Other Common Names:
Annual Chamomile, German Chamomile, Scented Mayweed, Hungarian Mayweed

Chamomile is used as an herb tea, commonly known from the story of Peter Rabbit, whose mother gave him tea made with it for his stomach ache. An annual herb native to eastern and southern Europe, chamomile grows well in zones 3–7, in fertile, well-drained soil with a pH of between 5.6 and 7.5. It prefers full sun, or part shade in areas where the sun is intense. It grows well in cool temperatures but subsumes to hard frost – the name of the game is not too hot, not too cold. Chamomile grows fine in a pot or other container, including a wall garden.

The small, daisy-like flowers bloom from early- to mid-summer and continue through to frost, especially if kept harvested or deadheaded. The flowers have a strong, fruity smell that is often apple-like. The Spanish name is manzanilla – little apple. A second herb, *Chamaemelum nobile*, that is used the same way as annual chamomile, is hardy in zones 4–9 but has flowers that are more bitter. This plant is a low-growing perennial called Roman chamomile. Annual chamomile is also closely related to pineapple weed (*Matricaria discoidea*), sometimes called wild chamomile, but that species lacks the white petals around the yellow true flowers.

Propagation

Seeds are tiny but easy to grow. Plant in place in the ground or in a pot, pressing firmly into the soil. Don't bury them, as they require light, and they will germinate in one to two weeks. Chamomile is not particular to type or pH of soil. It self-sows if the seed is allowed to ripen. Transplant seedlings about eight inches apart. Don't try to move full-size plants of the annual type. The perennial type can be divided.

Keep flowers picked to encourage further blooming and prevent self-sowing. Remove dead plants once the annual variety is killed by the cold. Divide perennial herbs every three to five years.

Common Problems

Annual chamomile is susceptible to rust, powdery mildew, and other fungi in especially wet years, or if the soil is not well drained. Aphids are a known issue and larvae of a European moth (burnished brass moth) feed on it and can be an issue.

Medicinal Use

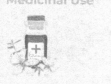

Chamomile has anti-inflammatory, antimicrobial, antispasmodic, mildly astringent and mildly laxative properties. It is most commonly used to make a water infusion (medicinal tea) to give relief from gastrointestinal issues, and as a mild sleep aid. The cooled infusion is used as a wash to soothe irritated skin with rashes, especially diaper rash, sunburn, scrapes, and insect bites. Chamomile can also be used for children, to relieve constipation in a gentle way. It may provide relief from monthly cramps and regular use of the tea has shown promise to slow or prevent osteoporosis.

Chamomile is used in many ways for pharmaceutical purposes. Several chemicals in chamomile essential oil have some antimutagenic and cholesterol lowering properties.

Safety

GRAS (generally recognized as safe) for most children and adults. Chamomile is from the same family as ragweed and may cause a reaction in those who have a known allergy. Use caution with this herb until you see how you react to it. While it is rare, large doses of chamomile may cause nausea and vomiting. It contains coumarin; be aware and test if you take regular medicinal doses along with drugs used to thin the blood. Your dose may need to be changed. It is recommended that you do not take chamomile at the same time as aspirin or other NSAIDs as it may interact with them.

Culinary use

The flowers are used in tea and certain soft drinks for their sweet, fruit-like flavor. The whole plant has been included in recipes for beer and ales, mostly by craft and home brewers. I even make jelly for my grandchildren with chamomile flowers; they love it!

Harvest the flowers as they open fully, which is every few days.

I've used chamomile in soaps, mouthwash, and cosmetics. The flowers are often included in potpourri or sachets for their sweet scent. In addition, dyes made from chamomile have a strong, warm yellow, gold or brown color, when used on protein fibers with an alum mordant. The color is pH sensitive.

Sometimes called English chamomile, the perennial type can be used as a lawn or between stepping stones in a walkway. Chamomile does not tolerate much traffic but can be very useful on slopes and in other hard to mow areas.

Sweet Annie

Family:
Asteraceae – Daisy Family

Botanical Name:
Artemisia annua

Other Common Names:
Sweet Wormwood, Annual Wormwood

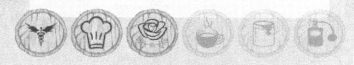

Sweet Annie is native to temperate Asia but naturalized in many temperate countries, including parts of North America. The leaves are dark green on top with a silvery underside, and are lacy and fern-like. Tolerant of poor, dry soil, this herb shows its appreciation for garden soil by growing taller. It has a pyramidal shape and often looks like a Christmas tree. It normally grows to a height of between four and six feet, but can get to eight feet when cultivated. Horses and cows won't eat it and you often find it growing in fields where everything else has been eaten. Sweet Annie is deer resistant.

It loves a sunny site but is not the least bit sensitive about soil fertility. It tolerates slightly acidic to alkaline soils as long as the soil is well drained. Grows well in zones 5–9. Sweet Annie prefers moderate temperatures and humidity but, as said before, this herb isn't particular.

Artemisia annua is an annual short-day herb. That means it doesn't develop flower stalks until triggered by the arrival of shorter days. The greenish-yellow flowers bloom in late summer and are very small, which makes it hard to see them.

Propagation

The seeds are tiny, even dust-like; that should tell you that they require light to germinate. Once four or so inches tall, you can allow the soil to dry out before watering. In short season areas, start seeds indoors six to eight weeks before the last frost date. I barely cover them, and I water by misting so the water doesn't push the seeds around.

This herb self-sows if allowed and often, once you grow it, you'll have it for years to come. It can become invasive if ignored for several growing seasons but weeds out easily. Transplants are hard to find but the seed is readily available in catalogs and online. Sweet Annie can take 7–21 days to germinate, depending on temperature. After they grow their second pair of true leaves, thin the seedlings to three feet (90 cm) apart.

Maintenance

I cut plants to the ground after they die. I also mark the area so I don't accidentally weed out the young seedlings before they're big enough to recognize. Sweet Annie has no common problems.

Medicinal Use

Sweet Annie has a long history of use in Chinese Traditional medicine as a hot water infusion to treat fever, inflammation, infectious diarrhea and malaria. Artemisinin, long considered the antimalarial component, is not water soluble. Another 'goodie' must also be antiviral and antiprotozoal because research shows sweet Annie tea works and it has been found effective to treat quinine-resistant malaria. This herb has many other phytochemicals. The highest concentration of artemisinin is in dried leaves taken from the top third of the plant (in new growth).

Safety

The same phytochemicals that give sweet Annie its medicinal value can also cause allergic reactions for some. The pollen of the blooming plant may cause a reaction if you suffer from hay fever. Those with ulcers or other gastrointestinal issues should not use this herb.

Other Uses

Often used as a sweet-smelling filler for fresh and dried arrangements. The blooming plants are quite stiff and make a wonderful wreath base that still smells sweet ten years later. My gardening gloves smell like sweet Annie even though I harvested mine over a year ago. The strong, but not unpleasant, smell repels insects and the herb has been used for hundreds of years in natural moth repellent sachets and blends. Isn't that amazing?

Harvest

For medicinal use, harvest the leaves of the upper half of the plant, starting three months after sprouting and as the leaves regrow. Depending on where you live, you should be able to get four or five harvests. For wreath bases, harvest after the flower stalks have stiffened. For scent, the oils will be strongest in the leaves when buds have formed but flowers have not yet opened; but honestly, this herb is strong enough to use for this purpose anytime the leaves are big enough.

Moth Repellent Sachet for Sock Drawer

4 parts sweet Annie leaves, dried and crumbled small
2 parts Lavender leaves, dried and crumbled small
1 part Clove buds, whole and dried
4 small bags with drawstrings or ribbons

Combine together and put one-quarter of the mixture into each of the four small bags. Tie or sew shut and place in desired drawer.

Purple Coneflower

Family:
Asteraceae — Daisy Family

Botanical Name:
Echinacea purpurea

Other Common Names:
Echinacea, Coneflower, Mad Dog

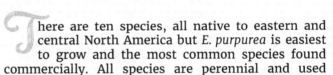

here are ten species, all native to eastern and central North America but *E. purpurea* is easiest to grow and the most common species found commercially. All species are perennial and used similarly, with *E. angustifolia* considered strongest but threatened and slower to grow, and *E. tennesseensis* and *E. laevigata* listed as endangered due to over-harvesting.

The large, showy flowers, borne on drought- and heat-tolerant plants, are valued for the flower garden and are often planted in the green areas of parking lots and in cities and other paved places. It always amuses me when I go to the local Cracker Barrel because they have them planted out front by the porch. The herb often reaches five feet tall when blooming and slowly increases in clump size as new roots form. It prefers poor, dry, even rocky, soils in full sun, unless growing in the more southern areas where the sun is strong. Then a bit of afternoon shade will be appreciated. It may bloom poorly in rich soil so go easy on the compost or other fertilizer.

Many cultivars and colors of *E. purpurea*, *E. angustifolia*, and *E. pallida* are now sold in greenhouses and garden centers. These cultivars were chosen for their beauty and are largely untested so if you want one for medicinal purposes, it is best to stay with the tested, unimproved species. The common name comes from the large seed cone that rises as the seed grows.

Propagation

To start purple coneflower from seed, plant in the late fall to provide naturally cold conditions, or stratify in the refrigerator for at least two weeks before planting. You will see seedlings come up in about two weeks. You can also propagate using vegetative methods, such as planting cuttings or dividing your plants, so that you keep specific cultivars pure, if that is important to you. Both root cuttings and division of clumps increase this plant.

Maintenance

You will find that coneflowers require little maintenance. Since they prefer dry soil, it takes a prolonged drought to need any water. I trim dead leaves and stalks after frost sends the plant dormant, unless I am leaving the seed cones for wintertime feeding of the birds. Remove empty cones before the herb breaks dormancy. You can divide the plants every three to five years if you're not harvesting the roots.

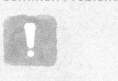

Common Problems

The biggest problem I've found may be Japanese beetles that show up here about mid-June, and can quickly strip a plant. I hand pick those into a container full of water. Powdery mildew, yellows, aphids, whiteflies , and mites can be issues for coneflowers and should be watched out for; these pests usually only occur in mass plantings such as commercial operations. Fungus can cause problems in poorly drained soil.

Medicinal Use

I always keep this in my kitchen for flu season. I use it in an immunity-boosting tea for my kids, who are able to go about their normal activities while all their friends are sick. This is because all species have immunity-boosting, anti-parasitic and antimicrobial properties. Purple coneflower has been found in studies to prevent respiratory illness but only has a small effect on viral illnesses. It is effective against bacterial infections and illnesses. Another interesting and important attribute it has is that coneflower has a positive effect on poisonous insect bites and snakebite.

Safety

GRAS for children aged 12 and older, and for most adults. One extensive study found that side effects were rare and limited to gastrointestinal issues and rashes. Check with your healthcare professional before taking medical amounts of any *Echinacea*, especially if you are taking other pharmaceuticals; there are possible interactions with medications used in treating common bleeding abnormalities, heart disease, and autoimmune issues such as lupus and psoriasis.

Studies have not found this herb to cause miscarriage

or birth defects but it is still not recommended for pregnant women. Be careful if breastfeeding as there have been an insufficient number of studies on the potential effects.

All parts of the plant are edible although the taste takes some getting used to, and so this herb has only been used as a survival food. The leaves and flowers are commonly used in teas.

Don't harvest the roots until at least the third autumn. It will take the herbs that amount of time to grow enough roots to ensure the herb continues after some root removal. It may take longer if you are growing one of the slower-growing species. The birds like the seeds so you may need to cover the cones so that some are left for you to use. Place a bag (I recommend a knee-high hose or stocking) over the seed cone and, once fully ripe, cut off and turn upright to shake and catch the released seeds. I harvest the leaves anytime before the flowering cycle, to use for my tea blends.

Sweet Goldenrod

Family:
Asteraceae – Daisy Family

Botanical Name:
Solidago odora

Other Common Names:
Licorice Goldenrod, Aaron's Rod, Woundwort.
Plus each species has its own common names.

Goldenrod herb naturally contains 7% rubber. It was the focus of Thomas Edison's experiments for a while and he bred a cultivar that had 12% rubber. Tires were actually made from this cultivar. Then synthetic rubber was invented, which was cheaper than using natural rubber.

Nana taught me the goldenrod blooms are the signal that summer is over and autumn has arrived. Sweet goldenrod (*Solidago odora*) is the preferred species for its taste, but any goldenrod is used similarly. There are over 200 species in the *Solidago* genus so at least one grows near you. The majority don't like soggy feet but a few grow in wet soil. All prefer the sun and hate the shade. Canada goldenrod (*S. canadensis*) is common in much of the northern United States. Other species have been intentionally planted and a few nurseries carry the hybrids.

Goldenrod is often unjustly blamed for causing allergies. The fact is that goldenrod pollen is heavy and spread by insects instead of the wind, making it highly unlikely to cause the symptoms of hay fever. You'd have to stick your nose into the flowers to make contact. Ragweed pollen is the usual culprit; this plant blooms at the same time as goldenrod and its pollen is blown about by the wind. Anything that you put on or in your body is capable of causing allergic reactions in susceptible individuals. Although allergy to goldenrod does occur, it isn't the problem most people think it is.

Sweet goldenrod grows to between two and four feet tall and has lance-shaped leaves and bright yellow flowers that bloom from late August through to early fall. A common 'weed,' it grows in fields, open areas, roadsides or near the edges of woods. Many species of goldenrod are the first plants to grow in abandoned land or after a fire. I walk out my door and see it growing everywhere. It's very popular with many pollinators as well, including butterflies and wasps (which are, in fact, surprisingly important pollinators).

Seed is very tiny and self-sows if allowed. Goldenrod slowly forms a clump, so division is the best way to increase a specific variety. Transplants are available, especially the hybrid varieties, in landscape centers and catalogs. With the popularity of planting native species, it's getting easier to find goldenrod.

Cut off flowers as they begin to fade. Not only does this improve the appearance of the herb, but it also prevents spread by seed. Cut dead plants to the ground after cold causes them to go completely dormant, and remove the dead foliage to prevent carrying mold or diseases over winter. Mulching plants after the ground freezes will help herbs stay dormant through false spring warm-ups, but this is a very hardy herb that doesn't require much help, unless you are trying to grow it outside its preferred zones.

The whole genus is host to several species of gall-causing insects. They do not harm the plant or limit its uses. Fungal or viral leaf spot may appear on lower leaves. Rabbits and groundhogs occasionally eat the herb, especially when first up and tender.

Goldenrod has been shown by studies to have diuretic, anti-inflammatory, and antimicrobial properties. It is used to reduce pain and swelling of wounds and infections, to prevent formation of kidney stones, relieve existing gravel, and ease eczema, hemorrhoids, arthritis and prostate enlargement. It is an effective remedy for upper respiratory issues, including seasonal allergy, sinus infection, colds and influenza and as a mouthwash for sore gums. In fact, I infuse it into my allergy specific elderberry syrup and my fire cider because it helps so much.

Goldenrod may cause an allergic reaction if the person is allergic to others in this same family. A very large dose may cause heartburn. This herb may cause high blood pressure to become worse, with its diuretic action, and this will cause sodium to become more concentrated in the blood. It may also cause dizziness if taken with other 'water pills,' by causing you to lose too much water. Be sure to check with your healthcare provider or pharmacist if taking allopathic drugs.

The flowers are edible and can be used anywhere that edible flowers are appropriate. The leaves may be cooked, like any pot herb (greens), while young and tender, or added to soups, stews and casseroles. This is another flower I commonly put into tea blends.

Dried flowers have been used as a wreath base and in dried arrangements. Use or freeze flowers at their peak for dye.

Young, tender leaves intended for culinary use may be blanched and frozen for winter use. I harvest aerial parts (everything from ground up) just as the flowers are ready to bloom. Harvest flowers for drying when they just start to show color. If you wait until the flowers are fully open, they will 'fuzz' when dried. You can still use them if they 'fuzz' but they aren't as good for tea that way.

To Make Goldenrod-Infused Oil

Fill a jar halfway with dried goldenrod flowers/leaves. Pour your preferred oil over the flowers until the oil reaches half an inch from the top. You can infuse the oil the slow way, the solar way or the speedy way.

- **Slow way** – Cap the jar and tuck it into a dark cabinet for 4–6 weeks. This method only works with dried herbs. Strain.

- **Solar way** – Don't cap the jar, but cover it with a piece of cheesecloth or scrap of old t-shirt instead. Set the jar in a sunny window for a few weeks. This must be done if using fresh herbs, as it allows the moisture to evaporate. The heat from the sun will help the oil infuse faster.

- **Speedy way** – This is especially good when making a large quantity of oil. Using a crockpot as a double boiler on the warm setting, heat for at least eight hours. This is nice because you don't have to watch it closely. As with the sun method, don't cap

the jar, but cover it with a piece of cheesecloth or scrap of old t-shirt instead. This must be done if using fresh herbs, but is optional if using dried herbs. Let the oil/herb combo sit overnight to cool, then strain.

- You can use the finished oil as is, or make it into a salve.

For the Salve:

3½ oz (100 g) goldenrod-infused oil

1/2 oz (14 g) beeswax

- Melt the oil and beeswax in a small pan that is placed in a slightly larger pan of water, to make a double boiler.

- Cool until skin starts to form and then stir until completely cool. This amount will fill three 2 fl oz (60 ml) tins.

Goldenrod-infused oil and/or salve is useful for muscle aches and pains and to prevent infection in minor cuts and scrapes. You can add more beeswax at small intervals if the consistency isn't to your liking.

Golden Oil

Common Barberry

Family:
Berberidaceae – Barberry Family

Botanical Name:
Berberis canadensis

Other Common Names:
Barberry, Allegheny Barberry, American Barberry.
This genus also includes the herbs blue cohosh
and mandrake that are not covered in this book.

American barberry (*Berberis canadensis*) is native to America, while a close relative, European barberry (*Berberis vulgaris*) – also called common barberry – is native to Europe but has been naturalized in much of the world. European barberry was brought to New England by British colonists in the 1600s. Barberry's popularity as a foundation shrub in the United States is due to the thorns it grows. One story that comes from Massachusetts is that the shrubs made British spies so uncomfortable that many colonists relied on them to help keep secret rebel plans a secret.

American and European barberries are hard to tell apart. Both are valued for their rich leaf color, spring flowers and easy care. They are both hardy, perennial, deciduous shrubs that are low maintenance and not the least picky about soil. Very tolerant of urban conditions, barberry can even be grown in containers. With pretty blooms and some kinds that have thorns (to stop peepers and the occasional spy), it's perfect for use as a foundation shrub. Also used to make a hedge, thanks to its uniform growth habit. Barberry grows to ten feet (3 m) high if allowed but can be pruned to keep it shorter. Flowers are yellow and form in long groups, called panicles, in the late spring. Berries ripen red in late summer or early fall. Barberry prefers normal soil moisture but is very drought tolerant once established.

American Barberry grows best in hardiness zones 4 –8, but there are a few that will thrive in zone 9 if given shade protection from the mid-day summer heat. A few rare cultivars survive in extreme climates like zones 3 and 10. This herb prefers full sun but tolerates even shade and is very adaptable to a wide range of soils as long as it drains well. The shrub has highly drought tolerance making it ideal for Xeriscape gardening.

Caution: The European common barberry (*Berberis vulgaris*) is illegal in four states in the USA. Japanese barberry (*Berberis thunbergii*) is illegal in 20 states in the USA as it is an alternate host for the black stem rust, a disease that can cause severe crop loss in grain crops. European barberry or barberries from various countries may be illegal in certain other countries as well ... when in doubt, check current law with your local agricultural agent.

Propagation

Barberry can be propagated by seed, but rhizome cutting is best for uniformity in a hedge. Seed requires eight weeks of stratification before moving to warmth. Herbs should sprout 30–35 days after moving. Cuttings are a little faster than seed. Birds love the fruit so it will need to be pruned after flowering to prevent them from spreading barberry.

Maintenance

Prune barberry after flowering if you wish to prevent spread by berry. If berries are desired for cooking, prune after harvesting those. Pruning before flowering will remove the buds and prevent flowering. Prune for height control anytime the plant is dormant. The plant is very tolerant of pruning. Best to transplant barberry after blooming or after the winter. Fertilizer is not usually necessary; mulch will aid in retaining moisture in dry weather.

Common Problems

Barberry has few problems but, especially in wet years, pests can include webworms, aphids, and verticillium wilt. There are wilt resistant cultivars. The thorns, although usually seen as a good thing, can cause physical harm under certain circumstances.

Medicinal Use

The medicinal use dates back more than 2,500 years. Berries are very high in vitamin C. Often used as an herbal tonic to stimulate appetite as well as treat gastrointestinal issues. The roots, rhizomes, and stems of all varieties contain the alkaloid berberine and can be used instead of the endangered and difficult to grow goldenseal (*Hydrastis canadensis*) for sore throats and many other infections. It is also used to relieve diarrhea, gastrointestinal issues and as an ingredient in many bitters.

Safety

GRAS for most adults in culinary and appropriate medicinal doses. Extremely high doses can cause nausea, vomiting or nosebleeds. In infants, berberine (the main medicinal constituent in barberry) may interfere with the liver's function to worsen jaundice. Internal use in medicinal amounts is not recommended if pregnant or nursing. Not enough studies have been done to say for sure, but berberine may interact with drugs meant to thin your blood, or with blood pressure medicines; check with your doctor before use.

Culinary use

Grown in many countries, barberries are very tart and made into jams, jellies and thirst-quenching punches. They are high in pectin and often added to low acid and low pectin fruits when making jam. One of the most popular traditional dishes in Iran, called *Zereshk Polo,* has barberry as its main ingredient alongside saffron and chicken.

Other Uses

Decorative uses are flowers in a bouquet. The stems and roots can provide a yellow dye to color paper but this has poor light fastness when used to color fabrics.

Harvest

Harvest stems in the late spring to all summer when the sap is flowing. Harvest berries when ripe, late summer to early autumn, and dry or freeze for out of season use. Dig roots in late fall to early spring (before breaking dormancy).

Zereshk Polo (Barberry Rice Pilaf)

4 cups Basmati rice, cooked
⅓ cup barberries
1 onion, large and sliced thinly
⅓ cup butter
½ cup sliced almonds
2 tablespoons sugar
¼ tablespoon orange peel, fresh and cut into thin strips with most of the white removed.
1 pinch saffron threads, crushed to powder and soaking in 1 tablespoon water

- Clean barberries well. They are harvested in a way that they contain small leaves, soil, and pebbles. Wash very well.

- Combine onion and butter in a large frying pan over medium-low heat. Saute until onions are almost caramelized (about 15 minutes).

- Add the almonds, sugar and salt. Turn heat up to medium and cook 5 minutes more.

- Add barberries, orange peel and saffron water. Cook, stirring, for 5 minutes more.

- Pour hot rice into a large serving dish. Pour barberry mixture over top and serve hot.

I know you are excited to try this and you SHOULD be! It's DELICIOUS. But this is just the tip of the iceberg ... you are about to find out about so many more medicinal and culinary herbs in this book.

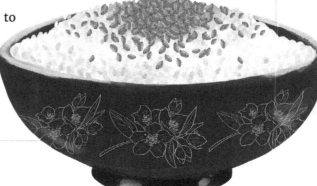

Anise-Hyssop

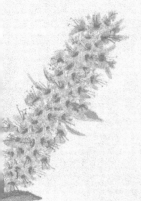

Family:
Lamiaceae – Mint Family

Botanical Name:
Agastache foeniculum

Other Common Names:
Elk Mint, Lavender Giant Hyssop, Blue Giant Hyssop, Fragrant Giant Hyssop

Anise-Hyssop is neither an anise nor a hyssop but got its name from the anise flavor of its leaves and the fact that it used to be in the hyssop family. Once proven otherwise, the name never changed. It is a short-lived perennial that grows between two and four feet (0.6–1.2 m) tall. It is native to North American prairies, dry fertile forested areas, plains and well drained fields in zones 4–9. Anise-hyssop prefers a pH of 6.0 to 7.0 but will tolerate soil a bit outside that range.

The foliage grows very straight, with fragrant leaves that are green on top and have short, whitish hairs on the bottom. The leaves have the smell and taste of anise. The plants prefer full sun, but will tolerate light shade. New growth has a purplish cast. All but seedlings are deer resistant as well as drought tolerant.

Ornamental yet scentless lavender-purple flower spikes appear, starting in June, and bloom continues until frost sends the herb dormant . The flowers provide nectar to hummingbirds, and attract pollinators and butterflies to the garden. It is a truly magnificent sight in full bloom! There is a cultivar with white flowers but its flavor is much diminished.

Propagation

The preferred form of propagation is by seeds that are planted indoors, 8–10 weeks before the last frost date. If started early enough, anise-hyssop will bloom the first year. The seeds are small so just barely cover them and they should sprout in 5–10 days. Plants self-sow readily and may become invasive if ignored, but undesired seedlings are easy to pull out.

Being perennial, this herb stays small for a long time, but much is happening underground. Plants usually don't get big until the second growing season and reach full size in the third. The herb forms clumps so division of an existing plant is effective. Transplants are available only at places that specialize in herbs. Space transplants 12 inches (30 cm) apart. The herb also grows well in large pots or containers that are at least eight inches (20 cm) wide. Indoors, give the brightest light possible.

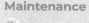

Maintenance

I prefer to deadhead flowers as they fade, to promote additional bloom and prevent self-sowing. But leave one or two flowers to ripen seed if transplants are desired. Cut dead plants to the ground after cold causes them to go completely dormant, and remove the dead foliage to prevent carrying mold or diseases over winter. Mulch plants after the ground freezes so herbs stay dormant through false spring warm-ups, until weather stabilizes for good.

Common Problems

Anise-hyssop is usually problem free. Young seedlings may suffer damage by slugs. Powdery mildew may be an issue in late summer with very humid or wet weather.

Medicinal Use

Anise-hyssop has diaphoretic, cardiac friendly and antioxidant properties. It makes a good-tasting internal treatment for cough, fever, digestive issues (including diarrhea), and as a poultice externally for wounds. It can also be used externally on minor burns. Tea is my preferred method of ingestion and it can be cooled for external use. Eight years ago, I brought this herb with us on a family ski trip to Vail and ever since then, my family demands anise tea on ski trips. It can also be infused into oils for salves.

Safety

Anise-hyssop is GRAS (generally recognized as safe) in culinary and medicinal amounts. The essential oil has been known to cause seizures, especially in susceptible people, so use caution until you know how it affects you and never use it undiluted.

Culinary use

The flowers make a pretty garnish and can be used anywhere as edible flowers, such as in salads, fruit salads, or baked goods. Bees make a light, fragrant honey from the flowers. The leaves are also edible and used as seasoning in salads, vegetables and certain meat dishes, desserts such as ice cream and cookies, teas, and syrups. Anise-hyssop has a natural affinity with peas and salmon. Commercially, anise hyssop essential oil is added for flavor to root beer liqueurs.

Other Uses

I love using fresh or dried flowers in arrangements and dried leaves and flowers can be added to potpourri for its strong, sweet anise scent. Many find it very attractive so it's often grown in a flower bed as a pretty backdrop flower in the middle or back of perennial borders, native or wildflower gardens, as well as herb gardens. As a companion plant, I have found that anise-hyssop repels cabbage looper moths and increases the harvest of horehound and annual chamomile.

Harvest

Tender young leaves may be harvested for fresh use all through the summer. Leaves to be dried for out-of-season or medicinal use are strongest when the flowers are just at full bloom, as the oil content in the leaves is the highest at that time. Flowers for tea or fresh use are best when three-quarters open.

English Lavender

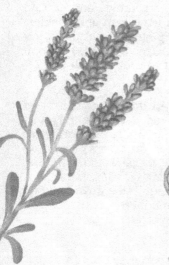

Family:
Lamiaceae – Mint Family

Botanical Name:
Lavandula angustifolia

Other Common Names:
Common Lavender, Narrow-leaved Lavender,
True Lavender

*L*avender is one of the most well-known herbs in all of history. It's seen in many myths, legends, folklore stories, and historical tales. It is even said that Cleopatra used lavender in her seductions and the asp, a venomous snake that killed her, was hidden among her lavender bushes.

Lavandula is a huge genus of over 47 known species, plus all the hybrids and various cultivars. *L. angustifolia* and its cultivars are the hardiest lavenders and known as English lavender, although they're not native to England. It's a subshrub (dwarf shrub) native to the Mediterranean area and grows best in similar conditions (well-drained, neutral to sweet soil). It likes good drainage so much, the herb may benefit from having gravel added to the soil in the area. English lavender will tolerate slightly acid soil but may be short-lived in it.

English lavender grows to two feet when blooming. Flowers are purple to pinkish-purple and form in spikes at the top of long stems. Like most herbs with a long history of use by humans, it has many cultivars; *L. a.* var. "Hidcote" and "Hidcote Giant," *L. a.* var. "Beechwood Blue," and *L. a.* "Imperial Gem" are a few. *L. a.* "Munstead," *L. a.* "Lady Lavender," and *L. a.* "Nana Rosea" are dwarf cultivars. In the following paragraphs, only the information after the other species' names pertain to them, while all other information is about English lavender.

Lavandula dentata (French lavender, Fringed Lavender) is native to the Mediterranean area and the Arabian peninsula. Plants grow 24 inches (60 cm) tall, and have gray-green leaves and purple flowers. French lavender will stand a dip to frost temperatures but not prolonged cold and it prefers alkaline soils.

Lavandula stoechas (Topped Lavender, French Lavender, Spanish Lavender) is sold in many landscape centers but is not hardy. Grow in a pot and take inside before cold weather in temperate climates. Winters over in zones 8–10. The flavor is harsher with more pine-like overtones. Usually used in air fresheners, insecticides, and for medicinal purposes.

Lavandula viridis (Green Lavender, White Lavender) is native to Spain and part of Portugal. This species has green leaves with white flowers. It's most often used for medicinal purposes because of the 51 different essential oils found in actively growing shoots. It doesn't tolerate cold temperatures.

Propagation

The first time I grew lavender, I did it with my kids and friend Olivia. We planted the seedlings and waited. And waited. And waited. We discovered the not-so-fun fact that lavender is slow to start from seed, taking one to three months to come up. Be patient, keep the area warm, and use a heat mat if starting in the spring. They don't need to be stratified. Seedlings stay small for a long time and won't bloom in the first year. It was worth the wait, though. Even the tiny seedlings smelled so wonderful. Softwood or hardwood stem cuttings of non-flowering tips are the usual way to propagate named varieties.

Maintenance

The best time to prune for shape and to stimulate new growth is right after lavender blooms, which is my favorite time when it comes to this plant because I save the pruned leaves and flowers for crafts or herbalism projects. If you don't harvest the flowers, deadhead them, especially the ones of repeat bloomers. Don't prune late in the summer. Lavender must be able to harden off new growth before frost.

Common Problems

Like all plants that need dry, well-drained soil, this herb suffers root rot if kept too wet. This has been my biggest hurdle with this plant, much to my dismay, because it's one of my favorite herbs. *Xylella* is a type of bacterium that causes disease in lavenders and also infects trees and shrubs; it is a problem for commercial growers but it can affect home growers too. The bacteria are native to the United States but have spread to Europe. It is spread from plant to plant by sap-sucking insects including spittlebugs. There is no cure. Control sap-sucking insects to prevent the spread of this disease, and remove affected plants to the trash or fire.

Lavender in medicinal quantities is used to relieve anxiety and promote sleep. Discontinue at least two weeks before surgery as when combined with anesthesia, it may depress the nervous system to dangerous levels. Lavender is often used to calm or prevent seizures, headaches, exhaustion and nervous issues. The essential oil, properly diluted, is added to massage oil to promote relaxation. I remember one particularly long day after college, one year during finals week. I got home and prepared an epsom salt and lavender bath mix. Let me tell you, there's nothing quite like relaxing in a lavender bath, with a cup of bedtime tea that has lavender in it as well, to just melt the day's stresses away.

Safety

Lavender is GRAS in culinary amounts. It's likely safe for internal use in medicinal amounts as well. Side effects to watch for are increased constipation, increased appetite, and possibly headache. When applied to the skin, lavender oil can cause a rash, although this is rare.

Culinary use

Dried flowers make a nice tea and are added to cookies, ice cream, and other desserts. The flowers are part of the classic French culinary blend known as 'herbes de Provence,' which is used to flavor cheeses, meats and vegetables. It is a staple in any of my relaxing or sleepy tea blends.

Other Uses

Lavender is added for scent to bath oils, lotions, and soaps. Flowers and leaves are dried and added to potpourri and perfume. Flowers in sachets are used to repel wool moths and add a nice scent to stored linens. It's also often used fresh or dried to add scent and color to arrangements, wreaths, and swags. I have sprigs of lavender in a wreath that I made ages ago, and they have continued to hold the lovely scent even after all this time; and the flowers have kept their beautiful purple hue.

Harvest

I do not recommend harvesting any leaves the first year. After that you may take up to two-thirds of the plant in mid-summer but I prefer to only take one-third of any herbs, just to stay on the safe side. Stop harvesting leaves early enough for the plant to recover before the cold comes; remember it's a subshrub and will not recover as fast as herbaceous herbs. Harvest flowers when two-thirds of the flower spike is in full bloom.

Horehound

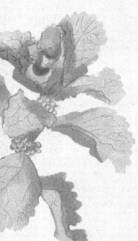

Family:
Lamiaceae – Mint Family

Botanical Name:
Marrubium vulgare

Other Common Names:
White Horehound

One summer I went to town and was only gone for an hour. When I got back my sheep had gotten through two fences (one around the sheep and one around my herb garden) and had eaten my chives, oregano, basil, coneflowers, scented geraniums, and everything else in my herb garden except my peppermint, rosemary, and horehound. I redesigned BOTH latches!

Native to temperate areas of Europe, Asia, and North Africa, and naturalized to North and South America, horehound has been spread world-wide by human activity. Horehound's natural site is dry, rocky, well drained soil in full sun. This perennial grows wild along roadsides and disturbed soils, even sandy soil. It's easy to grow, tolerating pH 4–8 soils and temperature zones 3–10. It has soft, grey-green leaves, with hairy upper surfaces and even furrier undersides, that can grow to two and a half feet (76 cm) tall and two feet (60 cm) wide. Like all mint family members, it has square stems, drooping leaves, and blooms, at leaf junctions, in dense spikes on the top third of each stem. The flowers are white and form in the mid-summer.

Horehound seeds are slow to germinate; that can be improved with stratification and use of seeds within three years. Seeds are tiny so plant on the surface with just a dusting of soil on top to prevent the wind from taking them. If you haven't the patience for seeds, divide a friend's plant or purchase a young transplant. Space or thin to about 12 inches (30 cm) apart and keep free from weeds. Horehound plants grow easily once established. Horehound is difficult to grow indoors without a greenhouse as it needs strong light, but young transplants will grow under artificial lights. Indoor plants may get spider mites.

Maintenance

Deadhead flowers as they fade, to promote additional bloom and prevent self-sowing. Leave one or two to ripen seed if transplants are desired. Cut dead plants to the ground after cold causes plants to go completely dormant and remove the dead foliage to prevent carrying mold or diseases over winter. Mulch plants after the ground freezes so the herbs stay dormant through false spring warm-ups, until weather stabilizes for good.

Common Problems

Deer, rodents and most other animal pests have to be very hungry before bothering the horehound as it's so bitter. Like most hairy/fuzzy plants, it is very susceptible to rot from too much water. There are no pests that are a problem. As a companion, it actually repels aphids and grasshoppers from the garden. If grown in a site that gets partial shade or in very humid years, powdery mildew can be a problem.

Medicinal Use

Horehound is used to relieve all breathing issues, including asthma, whooping cough, bronchitis, and swollen breathing passages. It is very effective for clearing congested lungs and is often used in cough syrups and cough drops. I recall my nana making us tea from her horehound and teaching me all about the plant. Now, I continue the tradition for my own family. Horehound is diuretic (increases urine production) and diaphoretic (causes sweating) which can break a fever.

This herb is often used to relieve digestive issues, such as indigestion, gas and bloating, diarrhea, constipation, and all gallbladder and liver ailments. Women have also used horehound to relieve painful menstrual periods.

Safety

Horehound is GRAS in culinary amounts. Horehound is likely safe for most people in medicinal amounts as well. It is NOT safe in large amounts or if you take allopathic medications to lower high blood sugar or high blood pressure. Horehound will have an additive effect and may lower either to dangerous levels.

Avoid this herb if you are pregnant or hoping to be pregnant as this herb causes uterine contractions and may cause loss of the fetus. Stay with culinary amounts if breastfeeding.

Bees are fond of horehound flowers and make nice honey from them. Horehound has been used as an ingredient in bitters for alcoholic drinks. It's also one of the bitter herbs used in the Passover celebration. A traditional hard candy is also made. This is another treat Nana introduced me to as it was, and remains, popular, particularly with the older generations. One of my great nostalgic joys is going into a small town general store and seeing horehound candy on the shelves.

Harvest

Plants don't usually blossom in the first year but you can still harvest a third of the top growth. After the plant has established its roots you can cut back to four inches (10 cm) when harvesting. Fresh herbs are used in ceremonies and can be made into tea. Dried herb is used in all infusions, syrups, capsules, pills, and cough drops.

Old-fashioned Cough Drops

- Bring two cups of water to a boil, remove from heat and pour over a cup of horehound leaves.

- Let steep till cool, at least 15 minutes.

- Strain to create a strong infusion. Measure liquid (tea) and use twice as much honey as tea. Mix together.

- In a 2 quart (2.2 liter) saucepan, add the honey mixture, 2 cups sugar, and 1/8 teaspoon cream of tartar. Heat over medium heat, stirring, until sugar is dissolved.

- Lower heat and continue cooking until the mixture reaches the hard ball stage. I use a thermometer to be sure but you can also drop a small dollop of mixture in cold water. It's done when it forms a hard ball.

- Pour candy into a well-buttered baking pan. Let cool just until you can cut candy into small squares and let it finish cooling. Once completely cool, dump out of the pan, breaking along score lines; then roll in powdered sugar to prevent the candies from sticking together. Store in a dry place, in an airtight container.

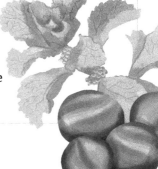

Spearmint

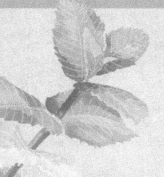

Family:
Lamiaceae – Mint Family

Botanical Name:
Mentha spicata

Other Common Names:
Tea Mint, Sweet Mint

Spearmint is native to Europe and southern Asia and is naturalized over most of the temperate world. It has a long history of use by humans. The first mention of spearmint is in the Bible, and it was also mentioned by the 1st century naturalist Pliny. Spearmint was introduced to Great Britain by the Romans, and to the United States by the first English settlers.

Spearmint has several subspecies and cultivars, including a curly-leaf variety (*M. s.* var. "Kentucky Colonel") that is used as a garnish, especially in such drinks as iced tea, mint lemonade, and mint juleps. It grows about 24 inches (60 cm) tall and has flowers that are white to light lavender.

All mints are perennials that are easy to grow and can take over the garden if allowed. They all grow best in partial shade with moist to wet soils but will tolerate full sun if well watered. Wild populations occur along rivers, creeks, ditches and moist hedgerows. Tolerant of a wide range of soils, these herbs spread by runners just under the surface of the soil. Some species are more invasive than others. Growth can be controlled by establishing plants in a large, bottomless pot or other container that is sunk into the ground. Leave an inch of rim sticking out above ground and cut off any runner that tries to escape over the edge. Or plant the spearmint above ground in a pot or wall garden.

There are many true mints with the same cultivation methods as above. Peppermint (*Mentha* x *piperita*) and its cultivar, chocolate mint, are more medicinal but are sometimes used for a pleasure tea. Peppermint has a cool-hot flavor that tastes of a York peppermint patty. The mints cross easily, making identification of unknowns difficult without DNA testing. However, known species and crosses include apple mint (*M. suaveolens*) that has a white variegated variety, Scotch mint (*M.* x *gracilis*), orange mint (*M. p. citrata*) and grapefruit mint (*M. p.* "Grapefruit") that has yellow variegation.

Propagation

Spearmint is easy to propagate from seed or, if you wish to keep the species or cultivar pure, you can propagate from stem or rhizome (root) cuttings.

Maintenance

Harvest before the seed sets to prevent self-sowing. Cut stems to the ground after frost sends the herb dormant. Rake up stems and add to a hot compost pile or put in the trash to control diseases.

Common Problems

Mints are susceptible to aphids, whiteflies, and spittle bugs. Many diseases affect mints but most of them are found in commercial fields with monoculture. Ones that may be found in home gardens are powdery mildew, verticillium wilt, and leaf spot. I've had spearmint in the same spot for over 50 years and the only issue has been spring spittlebugs, which may be remedied with a hard spray of water.

Medicinal Use

Spearmint is used for its antimicrobial properties. The essential oil of both spearmint and peppermint have been found to be more effective on Gram-positive than Gram-negative bacteria. The essential oil of both are added to toothpastes, mouthwashes and breath fresheners. In aromatherapy, spearmint is used to relieve post-anesthesia nausea. Mint oil can be rubbed on temples to relieve headaches and is drunk to relieve gastrointestinal issues, including gas, stomach cramps, and bloating, as well as to thin mucus. However, a small number of people are allergic to spearmint and may develop symptoms of diarrhea, heartburn or headache.

Culinary use

Spearmint is used in tabouli, curries, and seasoning blends. Makes a wonderful pleasure tea – iced or hot – and is also used in alcoholic drinks, like Mojitos and mint juleps, mint jelly for lamb and infused in milk for ice cream. The essential oil flavors gums, candies and other desserts.

Other Uses

Spearmint soaps are stimulating, helping you wake up in the morning, and the scent invigorates the brain to help workers and students perform better. My friend Jane loves to use it when she makes toothpastes and mouthwashes. Spearmint is sometimes used as a scent blender in perfume, potpourri and sachets. Many types of mints are added to cosmetics and make great smelling bath herbs, alone or in a blend. Mint oil is used as a natural insecticide for killing, wasps, ants, and cockroaches.

Harvest

Harvest Take up to two-thirds of the aerial growth when the herbs are at their strongest (just before, or just when a few lower flowers open on the spike). The oil content drops drastically after flowering. If you harvest in a timely manner, you may get a second harvest before the summer is over. All the true mints are best harvested thus. Use immediately or store for two days in plastic in the refrigerator; freeze or dry for later use.

Bee Balm

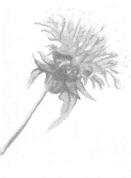

Family:
Lamiaceae – Mint Family

Botanical Name:
Monarda didyma

Other Common Names:
Bergamot, Horsemint, Oswego Tea

Bee balm has a tendency to grow all around here. You can find it in the fields, mountains, and on the roadside. It is said that the Native Americans used it in their bath water for rituals and the colonists made tea from it after the Boston Tea Party incident.

The genus *Monarda* is native to North America. The common name of bergamot refers to the citrus fragrance which is similar to the bergamot orange that is used to flavor Earl Grey tea. Bee balm has brilliant red flowers and blooming lasts about a month. The flowers are small but occur in a topknot-shaped bunch, making a glorious display. The plant prefers moist but well-drained soil and full sun but tolerates light shade and is hardy in zones 3–9. A close relative, wild bergamot (*Monarda fistulosa*), has pink or lavender flowers and is used in much the same way. Bee balm attracts hummingbirds and both *Monarda* species attract pollinators such as bees, butterflies, moths, and wasps.

Propagation

Bee balm starts easily from seed and has no special needs. Like most perennials, the plants stay small until their roots are set to survive winter and usually don't bloom until the second growing season; they reach full size only after the third. They spread slowly by creeping rhizomes so root cuttings or division also work well.

Maintenance

Harvest or deadhead to encourage blooming and prevent self-sowing. Cut to the ground once the cold sends the plant dormant.

Common Problems

This herb is susceptible to powdery mildew in humid conditions, especially if grown in a place with poor air circulation. Powdery mildew is a problem in humid areas, but usually not until after it has been harvested. The mildew doesn't seem to affect its ability to bloom but, left untreated, may cause loss of lower leaves.

Medicinal Use

Bee balm is antimicrobial, antispasmodic, diaphoretic and soothing. It is used to treat the symptoms of feverish colds and menstrual cramps, as a good mouthwash to treat mouth sores, sore throats, or infected gums, or as a wash for minor infections. Bee balm or wild bergamot is also used as a general stimulant.

Safety

Bee balm and wild bergamot are safe in culinary amounts. They are safe for most adults when taken as short-term medicine. Documented side effects are rare but watch out for heartburn, dizziness or muscle cramps. These herbs are considered unsafe to use in any but culinary doses, if pregnant or breastfeeding. The essential oil, even when diluted with a carrier oil, makes skin more sensitive to the sun. If using on your skin, cover up and use sunscreen to prevent burning. The essential oil is unsafe to use on children and in women who are pregnant or breastfeeding.

Culinary use

The flowers are edible and may be added to green, macaroni, or tabouli salads, plus they make a pretty garnish. Flowers may be frozen into ice cubes for a flavorful way to decorate cool, summer drinks. Both the leaves and flowers have a spicy citrus scent and flavor that make a fine tea. If you use only the flower bunches, the tea (hot or iced) has a gorgeous red color and will be appreciated as an addition to a family meal. My aunt Jeannie added lemon to bee balm to make a delicious jelly and always had everyone wanting the recipe. Leaves are sometimes used to flavor meats. Bees turn it into a nicely flavored honey.

Other Uses

The scent of both leaves and flowers blends well with rose and is often used in perfumes, potpourri and sachets. Bee balm flowers keep their scarlet red color when dried and both fresh and dry flowers have been used in arrangements, swags, and wreaths. The herb can also be used to scent a hair pomade (a substance used to style hair).

Leaves are best just before, or just as, the first few flowers open. Harvest flowers as they are in full bloom.

Common Catnip

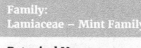

Family:
Lamiaceae – Mint Family

Botanical Name:
Nepeta cataria

Other Common Names:
Catnip, Catwort, Catmint (although this is usually reserved for a hybrid)

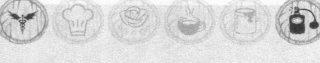

Catnip is attractive to two-thirds of the world's population of cats, including bobcats, jaguars, and other big cats. Whether or not a cat is attracted is hereditary. Catnip is native to the Middle East, southern Europe, and parts of China and Asia. It's now naturalized in much of the temperate world (hardy in zones 3–9). It's an easy-to-grow perennial, prefers full sun, and tolerates a wide range of soils as long as they are well drained. The fragrant flowers are usually white with an occasional plant that blooms pink; flowers appear in late spring and continue until frost, if not harvested.

There is a subspecies called lemon catnip (*N. c.* ssp. *citriodora*), that has a pronounced lemon scent. Another herb, known as *Nepeta x faassenii*, is a natural hybrid between *Nepeta racesmosa* and *Nepeta nepetella* and is often grown in a landscape just for its masses of attractive blue flowers. It has the common name Faassen's Catnip. The plant is perennial and not particular about soil type or fertility, is very drought tolerant, and still attracts cats. Both catnip and the hybrid known as catmint grow in the greenhouse or in pots outside but require strong light and get leggy when brought inside.

Propagation

Catnip is easy to start from seed and if allowed, will self-sow. Root cutting or division is used for named varieties. The seeds of catmint are predominantly sterile, but not completely, so propagation of the hybrid is mostly vegetative.

Maintenance

Harvesting and deadheading will encourage more flowers from catmint and prevent self-sowing by catnip.

Common Problems

Catnips have very few problems but if one is dying, a fungal disease is probably the problem. Ensure the soil is well drained, even though you have no control over the rain. You may have to resort to growing in a raised bed. Leaf spot or root rot may happen if catnip is grown in a site that has too much shade, too much water or is too crowded. All *Nepetas* are drought tolerant and deer resistant.

Medicinal Use

Most commonly used for its relaxing and sedative properties, catnip aids sleep and indigestion, increases appetite, and causes sweating if you want to break a fever. It is also used to relieve diarrhea. It is a traditional Italian medicine of one of my mentors, Gianna, who always suggests its use for infant colic, after having much success using it with her own children.

Safety

GRAS for most adults. Do be careful though, as if used with other sleep aids catnip may cause excessive grogginess. All catnips can induce uterine cramps causing possible loss of fetus. Avoid if you are pregnant or trying to become pregnant. Safe for use in children.

Culinary use

Catnip is sometimes used to flavor soups, stews, and sauces but more often flavors tea, other beverages, liquors, and table wines.

Other Uses

Catnip is used as a companion plant to attract lacewings and repel aphids or other bugs. Catnip essential oil in a spray has proven to repel mosquitoes, flies, termites, and cockroaches from the house. It doesn't work as well on skin.

Catnip may be harvested anytime after it is big enough but will be strongest just before, or when, the first few flowers are open. Cut two-thirds of the aerial herb and use immediately, or dry for later use. You should be able to get at least two harvests a summer.

How to Make Catnip Mice for Your Feline Friend

These are sachets stuffed with dried catnip, shaped like a mouse and used as a cat toy. You can draw eyes with fabric paint or embroider them on, but don't use buttons. They're easy to pull off and swallow. Also, sew the sachet shut, rather than just tying it, as catnip makes a real mess on the carpet. The mouse shape is nice but cats will play with a square, too.

Sweet Basil

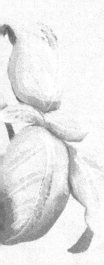

Family:
Lamiaceae – Mint Family

Botanical Name:
Ocimum basilicum

Other Common Names:
Sweet Basil

Summer before last, I planted my herb garden as well as a bee lover's flower mix. Once all were growing well, I realized that a few of the plants in my bee lover's mix area looked the same as my basil seedlings. Before long, I had so much basil that I took what I needed for my culinary and medicinal uses, and to share with family and friends, and still had plenty left to go to flower for the bees, butterflies, and other pollinators.

Sweet Basil is an easy-to-grow annual that loves the sun and heat, plenty of water and fertile but well-drained soil. The bright green leaves are a bit fleshy and go black at the slightest frost. The herb does survive in partial shade and indifferent soil, but the best flavor and regrowth is achieved in full sun and rich, well-drained soil. The plants grow well in most temperate zones for the summer but begin to suffer when temperatures drop to around 40°F (4°C) and can only be grown outside in the winter months in zones 10–11.

Flowers are white but a few cultivars have pink ones. They are small, almost insignificant, and occur in groups at the tips of the plant's stems. Flowering can cause a slightly bitter flavor to the leaf so it's best to cut the flowers off.

Basil will survive indoors but requires strong light to grow enough foliage to harvest; I recommend artificial light for 10–12 hours a day if you don't have a greenhouse. The plant will survive in front of a window but is very slow to regrow after harvesting.

Propagation

Seed is the easiest way to propagate basil. Transplant when nighttime temperatures stay around 50°F (10°C) or higher – basil really hates cold! Research your particular variety and allow as much distance between plants as the potential height of the plant. For example, if the plant will be three feet (90 cm) tall, allow 30–36 inches (75–90 cm) between seedlings. An exception is columnar basil, which grows mostly upwards and looks wonderful in a pot. Basil grows well in wall gardens, too. All the basils root easily and may be started in September to bring into the house or green house. Cuttings mature faster than seeds. Cuttings also root extremely easily and quickly in water as I learned happily after leaving some in water for a little too long one time, when I had harvested it for fresh use in the kitchen.

Maintenance

Water in dry weather when soil dries down to two knuckles' depth. Pinch or cut flower buds off as they form. Flowering will slow regrowth and basil dies if allowed to ripen seed. Allow the last flowers to remain if seed is desired. Top dress with compost in mid-summer after a harvest. Remove dead plants.

Common Problems

Fusarium wilt is the most common disease of sweet basil. Resistant cultivars have been developed for the greenhouse industry and they are now available for home use. Other issues that may affect basil are gray mold, mildew and bacterial leaf spot. Rabbits, groundhogs and other animals may feed on basil. Slugs, aphids, and spittle bugs can also damage the plants . Damping off can affect seedlings and bigger indoor plants, especially if kept too wet. Water from the bottom and allow the surface of the soil to dry between waterings.

Medicinal Use

Sweet basil has anti-inflammatory properties to reduce the development of, or improve, health issues that involve high levels of inflammation such as cardiovascular disease, diabetes, arthritis, and gastrointestinal conditions. It also has many vitamins, minerals, and antioxidants to fight the effects of stress, physical or mental, on the body.

Many of the health benefits contained in basil disappear during the drying process. Use fresh leaves to make tinctures, oils, and syrups. The essential oil has shown to have antifungal properties. A quick **Safety note,** Do not use this herb with other blood thinners.

Sweet basil has been used by humans for centuries; there are many cultivars as well as hybrids. Dark opal basil (*O. b.* "Dark Opal"), Genovese basil (*O. b.* "Genovese"), Thai basil (*O. b.* var. *thyrsiflora*), lemon basil (*O. b.* x *citriodorum*), and African blue basil (*O. kilimandscharicum* x *basilicum*) are a few.

Sweet basil is used in soups, vegetables, and casseroles. It has a natural affinity for anything made with tomato, making it a no-brainer for many Italian and Thai dishes. You can make canned tomato soup taste homemade by stirring in a little sweet basil.

There are several interesting chocolate desserts and ice creams made with milk that is first infused with sweet basil. The seed makes a gel when it comes in contact with liquid and that gel is used to thicken certain drinks. A popular cultivar, Thai basil, has a strong licorice scent.

Genovese basils are a group of cultivars that are generally regarded as the best for culinary use. They are commonly used to make pesto. The cultivar *O. b.* "Dolce Fresca" is a nice, mid-sized Genovese basil, while *O.b.* "Gecofure" and *O.b.* "Gemma" are cultivars that combine great disease resistance with good taste. There is now even a red-leaved Genovese basil (*O.b.* "Freddy").

Other Uses

In research, the essential oil has shown repellant and toxic properties towards mosquitoes. Before window screens, basil was grown in boxes or pots on a window sill to repel mosquitoes and flies. It still has value when people go camping.

Basil is often used as a blender in potpourri, sachets, soaps, bath herbs and other scented products.

The cultivar Tulsi, or Holy Basil, has religious significance in many religions including Greek, Romanian, Bulgarian, Serbian, and Macedonian Orthodox. And in Hinduism it's thought to be the manifestation of the Hindu goddess Tulsi.

Harvest

Regular harvest will encourage bushier growth and discourage blooming. If the weather is warm enough to allow steady growth, young plants are ready for the first harvest in about six weeks.

After harvest, basil can be kept fresh in a glass of water (bouquet style) in the refrigerator for about 3 days. Dried basil loses its flavor quickly so it is better to use it while fresh. A good method to preserve all that fragrant goodness for cooking, is to freeze it after blanching it quickly in boiling water. Best is to puree quickly in a blender or food processor after blanching, and freeze in an ice cube tray. To use, thaw a cube or two.

My Delizioso Pesto

There are many recipes for pesto, but this is the classic. Pesto can be used as a sauce for pasta, a dressing for salads and baked potatoes, or as a filling for star bread.

4 cups sweet basil leaves, packed

½ cup olive oil

2 garlic cloves

½ cup pine nuts

¼ to ⅓ cup parmesan cheese, grated

- Combine the first three ingredients in a food processor or blender. Blend until smooth, stopping to push down the basil as needed. Some say a blender makes a smoother sauce (but that's a matter of taste).

- Add the pine nuts and continue to blend.

- Add the cheese and blend until smooth.

- Use or store in a jar for up to 2 days, topped with olive oil, in the refrigerator. Using olive oil to seal out the air is an edible way to keep the pesto from turning black.

- Makes a great sauce for spaghetti or on pizza, and can be used as a dressing on a green salad. There are several baked goods that use pesto to their advantage, too.

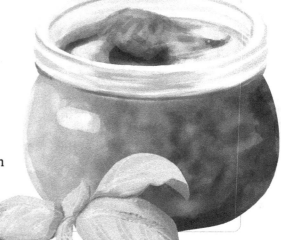

Oregano

Family:
Lamiaceae – Mint Family

Botanical Name:
Origanum vulgare

Other Common Names:
Wild Marjoram

*P*lants from this genus crossbreed easily, making it almost impossible to separate the oreganos from the marjorams without doing DNA testing. In practical terms, you need to taste the herb and if it has a bite, it's called oregano. If it tastes sweet and doesn't have a bite it is called marjoram.

Oregano prefers the hot, relatively low humidity and rocky, sweet soil of its native Mediterranean area. It receives plenty of rainfall but that drains away quickly. It will tolerate other areas but must have well-drained soil. Easy to grow, this is a beginner's herb that prefers a soil pH of between 6.0 and 9.0. Oregano grows well in partial shade but prefers full sun and the oils, and therefore the flavor, will be more intense when the plant is grown in the sun. The herb is about 10–24 inches (25–60 cm) tall when blooming. Flowers may be purple, pink, or white and they bloom in mid-summer (July and August in the Northern Hemisphere). If allowed, seed ripens in early autumn.

Greek oregano, also sometimes called Italian oregano (*O. v. hirtum*), is a very hardy cultivar that has a savory and earthy flavor and is considered the 'true' oregano. It grows best in zones 5–11. A staple of Italian cuisine, this herb is known best as 'the pizza herb,' brought back by soldiers who had served in southern Italy in WWII. It combines well with the spicy food that characterizes southern Italy. This very hardy oregano has white flowers .

Italian oregano (*O. v. virens* x *O. marjorana*) is another cultivar that is actually a natural cross that created a marjoram which is hardy in zones 6–9. This oregano is a bit milder than the Greek one and is preferred in northern Italian cuisine, along with sweet marjoram.

Propagation

Oregano seed starts easily but if you want a specific cultivar, you'll need to buy a transplant, or get a stem cutting, or possibly a division, from a friend. Seedlings need a little attention, mostly watering, but once established, they thrive on being ignored. Too much attention is the easiest way to kill oregano. Especially if grown in a pot, let the soil dry out to at least two knuckles deep before watering.

Common Problems

Aphids and spider mites are a couple of issues you may encounter when growing oregano. They can generally be easily controlled with a strong water spray that knocks them off the plant but the use of neem oil or other insecticide may be needed for infestations. Leaf miners, the larvae of black soldier flies, are another possible concern. Since they feed on the inside of the leaves, leaving tan or brown trails in their wake, insecticides won't work for them. The leaves must be removed from the plant and destroyed. Diseases that might cause problems are rust (remove the affected leaves) or root rot (rarely cured and plants usually need to be destroyed).

Medicinal Use

Oregano has antimicrobial, antioxidant and anti-inflammatory properties and is used for treating health issues that have these as part of the picture. These include conditions such as UTIs, athlete's foot, influenza, diabetes, infections and even certain cancers. It is used to lower LDL cholesterol, improve gastrointestinal health, and treat heart disease.

Sixty different compounds have been identified in oregano essential oil, extracted from the leaves, and this is why the oil can be used to treat many ailments. You can't make your own essential oils without a still (a setup of equipment used to capture and distill the plant's essential oils), but infused oil is the next best thing. It can be used in similar ways to essential oils that have been diluted with a carrier oil.

Culinary use

Apart from flavoring pizza, oregano is found in cucumber and tomato dishes, including marinara sauce used for spaghetti and lasagna, meats (especially barbecue and shish kabobs), vegetables, and casseroles. Oregano flowers are also edible, and are used in salads and as a decorative garnish. A very dear friend of mine, Dora, is second generation Italian/

American and her mother, who is full blooded Italian, always says (in her wonderfully strong accent, even after living for over 40 years in the United States) that no spice cabinet is complete without oregano.

Oregano has an intense flavor. Good-quality oregano may be strong enough to almost numb your tongue, but cultivars adapted to colder areas often have less intensity. Factors such as climate, season, and the soil it's grown in affect the aromatic oils present and, over the years, many cultivars have been developed. Some are more bitter, sweet, or peppery than others.

Harvest

Oregano can be harvested when needed but is at its strongest, for drying and medicinal use, just before flowering. It's best to cut it to the ground as oregano gets bitter after blooming. The herb will regrow, giving you a second harvest. Cutting also serves a second purpose: it will prevent ripe seeds from developing. Plants grown from these seeds will be inferior to plants rooted from cuttings.

Surprise Infusion Recipe

To make an infused oil, fill a jar half full of dried oregano leaves and fill to about half an inch from the top with oil of choice. Allow to infuse for four to six weeks in a warm, dark place. Strain and use or store, sealed tightly, in a cool, but not cold, dark place.

Garden Sage

Family:
Lamiaceae – Mint Family

Botanical Name:
Salvia officinalis

Other Common Names:
Common Sage, Dalmation Sage, Culinary Sage, Kitchen Sage

Garden sage is a woody subshrub that everyone should grow. An old saying often repeated by herbal practitioners is 'Why should a man die when sage grows in his garden?' In folklore, this herb is associated with longevity and immortality. The gray-green, slightly fuzzy leaves and early to mid-summer purple flowers are attractive. The bush gets to 24 inches (60 cm) tall and becomes just as wide, unless clipped shorter. Native to southeastern Europe, sage is evergreen in most climates, and hardy in zones 5–9. Common sage tends to be hardier than most cultivars. All prefer warm, well-drained locations and neutral to slightly acidic soil. None likes extreme climates. All grow well in pots, window boxes, and wall gardens.

Cultivars can have white, pink or purple flowers that appear in late spring and early summer, as well as cream, yellow, purple or rose-colored leaves. One cultivar, called tricolor sage, has white, rose and purple variegated leaves. The cultivar known as *S. o.* "Berggarten" has large leaves but rarely blooms, while *S. o.* "Purpurea" has purple leaves. Pineapple sage (*Salvia elegans*) is a close relative. It is a tender perennial with leaves that really smell like pineapple, and gorgeous red flowers that are triggered to bloom by the short days of late summer. Sage needs strong sunlight when grown indoors.

Propagation

The large seeds are very easy to start and grow quickly. Cuttings root easily and are the best way to propagate specific named cultivars.

Maintenance

Remove any winter damage or dead branches in the spring. A spring side dressing of compost is usually enough fertilizer. Never cut plants to the ground. Don't cut plants at all in the first year. After that, cut back or harvest by two-thirds when sage starts to open flowers; the flavor is strongest and it will encourage new growth. Old stems get woody. Replace plants every four or five years. Water when soil becomes dry at a depth of two knuckles.

Common Problems

Sage has few problems in well-drained soil. As with most drought-tolerant herbs, root rot can be a common problem in wet years or if watered too often. Slugs, caterpillars, and spittle bugs can be an issue and spider mites or white flies as well, if air is dry. I have occasionally had issues with caterpillars. I just hand picked them off my sage plants. I prefer to do this rather than spray them with anything toxic like neem oil, but I am willing to do this rather than lose my plants.

Medicinal Use

Sage has high antioxidant and anti-inflammatory properties and is used to relieve gastrointestinal issues such as gas, heartburn, stomach pain and loss of appetite. This herb also helps treat memory loss, Alzehiemer's dementia and depression. When sage is powdered and added to baking soda it can be used to brush and whiten teeth, and the same mixture reduces perspiration when used as a deodorant. It helps to reduce milk supply when weaning, reduces hot flashes, and relieves painful periods. Cooled infusion is often used on sunburn, as a gargle for sore throats and gums, or on cold sores. Sage is under investigation to lower total and LDL cholesterol and triglycerides. I recently made a mouthwash for my husband out of infused oils, including sage essential oil, for a severe toothache while we waited on a dentist appointment. It was such a big help.

Safety

GRAS in culinary amounts. Safe in medicinal amounts for most adults and older children. Do not use sage internally on infants or young children. Large doses may cause seizures or rapid heart beat. Use with caution until you see how it affects you. Because of its ability to reduce milk supply, be cautious when breastfeeding unless that is the effect you are looking for.

Sage is used to flavor soups, eggs, sausage and poultry and is an ingredient in commercial poultry seasonings. American Thanksgiving stuffing wouldn't taste right without sage. It is used to flavor vegetables, like mashed potatoes, butternut squash or sweet potatoes. Minced fresh sage is added to biscuits, rolls and breads, honey and herbed butters. It is also a common ingredient in a delicious Italian seasoning mix.

Other Uses

Sage makes an attractive base for wreaths and can be used fresh or dried for arrangements. Used as a dye for dark hair, and greens or yellows, depending on mordant, or grays with iron on natural textiles. Sage is also used by Native Americans for smudging as well as by other cultures and religious groups for cleansing the air. My aunt makes the most beautiful dried sage bundles and adds other herbs such as lavender or rosemary to use in her own spiritual practices. The scent that the bundles release as they burn is positively amazing.

Harvest

Sage has the strongest constituents and flavor just before, or when, first flowers begin to open. Use immediately, store in the refrigerator for up to three days, or dry for use out of season.

Rosemary

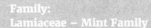

Family:
Lamiaceae – Mint Family

Botanical Name:
Salvia rosmarinus

Other Common Names:
Anthos, Compass Plant

This herb had the botanical name *Rosmarinus officinalis* until 2017 when DNA testing proved it to be in the *Salvia* genus. It is an evergreen shrub with needle-like leaves, native to the Mediterranean region and with a long history of human use. Rosemary can survive severe droughts making it perfect for xeriscapes. A cultivar, named after Arp, Texas, is said to be much more hardy than others. It is hardy in zones 7–10.

It still may die from the winter cold in Ohio. I have been told by gardeners from Idaho that it often survives winter there, although it sometimes dies to the ground, only to sprout again from the roots in the spring. I think it's because Idaho's snow lasts until spring, protecting the shrub underneath, while the snow in Ohio falls and melts, with up and down temperatures which are sometimes below zero but frequently there is no cover. Mulch may help it to survive short, cold spells but not extended ones.

Rosemary does best in well-drained soil with a pH that is neutral to slightly alkaline (7–7.8). The shrub can live 25 to 30 years. There are many subspecies and cultivars. Some are upright and some are prostrate. The upright ones can reach six feet (1.8 m) in height and are often used as aromatic landscape shrubs in areas with mild winters. Trailing varieties look pretty over retaining walls, in window boxes, and wall gardens. All grow well in pots, greenhouses and wall gardens. If grown inside, they require strong light or they become weaker as the winter goes on.

Rosemary has white, pink, blue or purple flowers, depending on the cultivar. The plants flower almost continuously in warm areas or if grown inside; they bloom from late spring through the summer when grown outside in temperate climates. There are few things as pretty as a tall rosemary shrub covered in blue flowers. A few popular cultivars are *S. r.* "Albus" with white flowers, *S. r.* "Majorca Pink," which is an upright form with pink flowers, and *S. r.* "Tuscan Blue," an upright form with blue flowers. *S. r.* "Lockwood de Forest" is a prostrate form with blue flowers.

Propagation

Rosemary is very slow from seed, both with a low germination rate and slow growth the first year. The preferred method is rooted stem cuttings and vegetative methods are necessary anyway to perpetuate named cultivars. Buy transplants, especially if you're not yet able to root successfully or only want one specific type. The herb is tolerant of clipping for shape and is pruned into topiary, knot gardens, or low hedges.

Maintenance

Remove any dead branches or damage after weather stabilizes in early spring. Trim for harvest and shape as needed. Water when dry but be careful not to overwater. Water pots from the bottom. Rosemary requires strong sunlight indoors and can be difficult to keep healthy and growing in the winter if you don't have a greenhouse.

Common Problems

Due to the high oil content, rosemary usually isn't bothered by much. It may develop mildew in humid weather, and root rot in wet conditions or if not well drained. Damping off fungus may kill seedlings and you will need to watch for blight. Aphids, spider mites, spittle bugs and scale are a few pests that may be an issue.

Medicinal Use

Rosemary has antimicrobial, anti-inflammatory, and antioxidant properties. Compounds in rosemary lower blood sugar levels, reduce anxiety, and improve digestion. It has shown promise against certain cancers and is said to slow age-related macular degeneration. The essential oil is rubbed on temples to fight headache, improve concentration, and support aging brains.

Safety

Rosemary is GRAS in culinary amounts. Medicinal doses are generally regarded as safe for most adults. Very high doses may cause nausea and vomiting, uterine bleeding, and kidney irritation. Rosemary contains a chemical similar to aspirin and so may cause an allergic reaction in those sensitive to aspirin or salicylates. Do not use medicinal amounts with bleeding disorders or if taking a drug designed to thin the blood. Also avoid this herb if you have a seizure disorder, and don't use rosemary in quantities other than culinary doses if you are pregnant or nursing.

Undiluted essential oil is not safe. Even when diluted it can cause rash and sun sensitivity. Cover up and use sunscreen if you have applied rosemary essential oil.

Culinary use

Rosemary leaves are used as tea and to flavor meats, stuffings, and vegetables. Also used in table mustard, salad dressings, herb butters and breads, and in seasoning blends. Rosemary has also been made into a jelly and added to shortbread cookies.

Other Uses

Rosemary extract has been shown in research to prevent rancidity in oils, soaps and natural cosmetics.

The leaves are often burned as incense or included in potpourri and sachets, as well as used to brew a hair rinse for dark hair. Rosemary branches make fragrant wreath bases or are used, fresh or dry, in arrangements or garlands. The essential oil is used in cleaning products, air fresheners, perfumes, bath oils, and shampoos. On textiles, rosemary dye can give from a buttery yellow to an olive-green color. This herb is considered sacred by many cultures who often use it as an herb for remembrance. An Egyptian friend of mine, Aharon, recently lost his grandfather. They made sure they used rosemary in the funeral especially given how much his grandfather loved this herb and its many uses.

Harvest

Rosemary is best harvested when at least three months old and actively growing in late spring through early summer. The flavor of this herb is strong enough to harvest whenever needed but is strongest when the plants are just starting to bloom.

Remember, this is a shrub. Do not cut off more than one-quarter of the length of the branches at any time. Be sure to stop harvesting in time for new growth to harden off before freezing temperatures arrive; new growth is tender. Use immediately, keep for several days in the refrigerator, or freeze or dry for later use.

Thyme

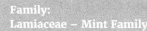

> **Family:**
> **Lamiaceae – Mint Family**
>
> **Botanical Name:**
> *Thymus vulgaris*
>
> **Other Common Names:**
> English Thyme, Common Thyme, Garden Thyme,
> French Thyme, Summer Thyme

Thyme is a perennial, evergreen subshrub about 12 inches (30 cm) tall, from the Mediterranean area. It needs conditions found there; plentiful water yet very well-drained soil, neutral to a little on the alkaline side, and full sun. Thyme suffers rot if the soil doesn't drain well but is very drought tolerant. Being a subshrub, it doesn't recover from damage or harvesting as fast as many other herbs. It gets about 16 inches (40 cm) wide, reaching full size in its third growing season. Thyme blooms with pinkish-white to pinkish-purple flowers from early summer to frost.

Like so many herbs with a long history of human use, *T. vulgaris* has many cultivars that vary by leaf shape, including French, German, and English versions. Some of the most commonly grown species and cultivars are lemon, lime, and orange cultivars (*T. citriodorus* varieties), caraway thyme (*T. herba-barona*), creeping wild thyme (*T. serpyllum*), and mother of thyme (*T. praecox*). All the thymes grow well in pots and other containers, window boxes, and wall gardens. Pollinators love feeding off all the different varieties of thyme.

Propagation

Thyme starts easily from seed but stays small for a long time. It roots from stem cuttings, layering and division. The vegetative methods are best for propagating named cultivars as there is too much unpredictable variation from seeds.

Maintenance

If not harvesting, deadhead the spent flowers to encourage new ones. Don't cut down in autumn or winter as new leaves come from existing stems. Prune off any winter damage in late spring, when the herb is actively growing. Spring composting is usually all the fertilizer that it needs.

Thyme is not bothered by many pests. Aphids and spider mites may occur. Rot and other fungal diseases might occur if you have a very wet year, especially in the winter, when damage accumulates.

Medicinal Use

Thyme and the essential oil of thyme contain large amounts of thymol and are very antiseptic and antimicrobial. It's used in toothpastes and mouthwashes, and in face washes to fight acne. Thyme makes a good wash for cuts, scrapes and rashes to prevent or treat infection. Used in a neti pot (which is a nasal irrigation device), the cooled water infusion can aid a sinus infection. Thyme infusion can also be used as a gargle for sore throats or a drink to assist with coughs, colds and bronchitis. It is used to boost general immunity, and to lower cholesterol and heart rate. A mentor of mine, Cathy, swears by a thyme cough syrup that she makes regularly, especially during the winter season. Since trying it for the first time a couple of years ago, while fighting off a serious upper respiratory infection, I am a believer in it as well and it's now a must have in my apothecary.

Safety

Thyme is GRAS when used in culinary amounts. It is also safe for most adults when used in medicinal amounts for a short time. The side effect of gastrointestinal upset has, however, been reported by a few users. Large amounts of thyme may increase clotting time, so don't use it with drugs intended to thin your blood. Stop using thyme two weeks before surgery. Avoid medicinal amounts when pregnant or if you have a health issue made worse by estrogen exposure.

Culinary use

Thyme is an ingredient in many spice blends including za'atar, which is used in Middle Eastern and Mediterranean cooking. It goes well with most meats (especially beef), vegetables and cheese. Large areas of Malta and Greece are covered with wild thyme which the bees use to make wonderful honey.

Thyme infusion makes a good general disinfectant to clean counters, use in the laundry, or as a rinse for dishes when someone in the house is ill. It kills mold on walls and other woodwork and is used to repel mice and rats.

Harvest Harvest when big enough and when needed. As a subshrub, it won't recover as quickly as some other herbs. Take only a third of the plant and stop harvesting in time for new growth to harden off before freezing weather arrives.

Thyme Cough Syrup

1 cup honey
1 cup extra virgin olive oil
2 lemons, sliced
¾ cup fresh thyme, rosemary, and/or sage, or ½ cup dried herbs
1 inch ginger and/or turmeric root, grated
5–8 garlic cloves, minced

- Place all ingredients, except honey, in a saucepan on low heat. Infuse for 30–45 mins.

- Remove from heat and let cool. When cooled, strain and mix well with honey.

- You can store it in the fridge for 3 months or on the countertop for about 45 days. Take a tablespoon at a time as needed.

Apothecary Rose

Botanical Name:
Rosa gallica var. officinalis

Other Common Names:
French Rose, Gallic Rose, Rose de Provins

*I*s there any flower more abundant in sensory overload than a rose? Good looks, delicious scent, wonderful for cutting, food, and medicine, few perennials can stop you in your tracks like a rose in full bloom.

The apothecary rose has been cultivated as an ornamental for centuries and used as medicine for millennia. The ancient Greeks believed that the goddess of love, Aphrodite, named the rose in honor of her son Eros, the god of love. It was described by ancient Greek poet Sappho as 'the queen of flowers' in about 500 BCE. The red rose has been used to symbolize romance and love ever since.

The apothecary rose is native to ancient Persia in the part of the world that is now Iran and Afghanistan. Crusading knights brought it back from the Middle East to Europe along with other 'discoveries.' The rose was known in Europe before 1310 and every European medical herb garden in a monastery or convent had at least one. In England, the apothecary rose was adopted by the House of Lancaster, with the rival House of York choosing a white rose; and the ensuing War of the Roses is well known.

This deciduous, perennial shrub has a nice form that grows three to four feet (90–120 cm) tall and four to six feet (120–180 cm) wide, with gray-green foliage. The rose grows in zones 4–8 but is iffy unless protected in zone 4. Although it prefers full sun, it is one of the roses that can tolerate light shade and still bloom. Its branches are thickly covered with thorns. Provide good air circulation and avoid overhead watering to prevent much disease. This rose is appropriate for borders, cottage gardens, low hedges and large containers.

The flowers are exceptionally fragrant, three to four inches (7–10 cm) across, dark pink to light red (depending on how you see color) and semi-double, with dark yellow centers. The blooms are prolific, almost covering the foliage. Unlike modern hybrids, this rose only blooms once in the late spring but for a decently long period of about four weeks. Like most roses, although it prefers rich organic soil, it will tolerate poor soil as long as it drains well. Be careful of your soil's nitrogen level or you may get leaves at the expense of this year's flowers. The fruit of the rose is a berry-like structure called a rose hip that ripens orange to brownish. Hips are very rich in Vitamin C; among the richest sources of any plant. The hips are eaten by people, animals, and frugivorous birds.

Propagation

Propagation is by softwood cuttings, semi-hardwood cuttings, hardwood cuttings, grafting or budding. The usual way for home increase is by means of softwood cuttings. Commercial plants are usually grafted onto a root stock to prevent suckering. The apothecary rose is sometimes available where old (aka heritage) roses are sold, or by mail order.

Maintenance

This rose is extremely healthy, tough, and reliable, as roses go. Cut any dead or dying canes away in the spring and remove any suckers to control width, if a grafted plant was not chosen. This rose does not usually need pruning but annual pruning for shape, if done, should be done right after blooming and no later. The apothecary rose blooms on old wood that was formed the previous year and if you prune later, you will be cutting off the flowers. Do not deadhead or you won't get any hips. You can pull off petals one by one, leaving the center, and thus harvest both.

Common Problems

Roses can be a bit of a challenge to grow, depending on where you live. Even so, I highly recommend growing the apothecary rose as it is well worth the trouble. All roses are prone to powdery mildew and black spot. These problems have their own chapter as there are organic controls. They will be a particular problem in wet years or in areas with a humid summer.

There is also a tiny mite (called an eriophyid mite) that spreads a virus causing rose rosette disease. This disease causes the rose to grow strangely deformed stems, leaves, and flowers. These mites are so small they can be seen only under strong magnification and are spread by the wind. The host for the virus is usually the multiflora rose, which has been reported as growing in all but nine states and three provinces in North America. There is no cure or treatment – yet. If you have a rose with this disease, remove all of it, even the roots, to prevent spread of both virus and mite. Do not plant another rose in that area for several years.

Medicinal Use

The apothecary rose was first valued for its strongly scented petals that, even when dried, have medicinal qualities. Rose petals are mildly sedative, antiseptic, astringent, anti-inflammatory, and antiparasitic. They are also high in antioxidants. They can be used as a mild laxative, a good supportive tonic for the heart, and are great at lowering LDL cholesterol.

The antiseptic nature of rose petals makes them a wonderful treatment for wounds, bruises, rashes and incisions. Rose water packs a lot of hydration to the skin. Its antioxidant and antibacterial properties improve the skin's barrier and reduce transdermal water loss. Because of this, it shouldn't trigger the sebaceous glands to pump out extra oil to accommodate overly dry skin. Rose water is especially hydrating when combined with other moisturizing ingredients, such as ceramides or glycerin. These help to moisturize the skin, protect the skin barrier and prevent further water loss from the skin.

Rose seed oil is pressed from the hips of a related type of rose and is used in many salves and cosmetics that treat eczema, acne, scars, stretch marks, and discourage the development of wrinkles.

Safety

Rose petals are generally regarded as safe. Under the American Federal Food, Drug, and Cosmetic Act, there are only certain *Rosa* species, varieties, and their parts, that are generally recognized as safe (GRAS); these include *Rosa gallica* and varieties of this species. The laxative properties are so mild that the rose is considered safe for use in infants. Due to their high vitamin C content, rose hips can cause diarrhea, but this requires the consumption of a really large amount.

Culinary use

Rose-flavored syrups, drinks, jams, cookies, vinegars, candies (including candied rose petals), and frozen desserts such as ice cream, are popular. Rose creams (rose-flavored fondant covered in chocolate, often topped with a crystallized rose petal) are a traditional English confectionery widely available in the UK. Rose hips are made into jams, jellies, soups, muffins, and breads. Both rose petal tea and rose hip tea are great hot drinks for those wanting or needing to avoid caffeine.

Other Uses

Rose perfumes are made from rose oil (called attar of roses), which is a mixture of volatile essential oils obtained by steam distilling the crushed petals of roses. An associated product is rose water, which is used for cooking, cosmetics, medicine and religious practices.

Rose petals are a common base for potpourri or sachets, with many recipes abounding. Rose petals were simmered in a cast iron pot until black and then rolled into beads. When dry, they were strung into rosaries, as the name refers. The warmth generated by handling the beads released their fragrance.

Dry rose petals have also been added to non-tobacco smoking blends.

Harvest

Leaves are most fragrant when buds have formed but not yet opened. Pick flowers as they open. Hips are picked when fully ripe, usually just before, or just after, frost in most areas where roses grow. You may have to cover the hips to beat the birds to them. I use old knee-highs or pantyhose.

The simmering method is the easiest and quickest way to make rose water, which is useful for cooking, medicine, and cosmetics.

Six roses
Distilled or filtered water
A large pot
A nut milk bag or strainer
Measuring cups
Sealed container (jar or spray bottle)

1. Remove the petals from the stems until you have 1 cup of fresh petals. Remove any bugs you find while pulling the petals from the stems.

2. In the pot, submerge the petals in just enough water to cover them, about 1½ cup. Any more will make the rose water too dilute.

3. Bring the pot of water to a simmer. Once the mixture starts simmering, cover and reduce heat to low. Leave for 15–30 minutes or until the petals have lost most of their color.

4. Turn the heat off, leave the lid on and allow it to cool completely.

5. Strain to separate the petals from the rose water. Using a nut milk bag gives the best color but a strainer will also work. When you're done, add the petals to the compost; almost all of the color and fragrance is gone.

6. Place rose water in a sealed container. Keep a small bottle for culinary use or add to your favorite cosmetic, including rose water and glycerin hand lotion. It can be kept as is in the refrigerator for up to a month, or in your bathroom cabinet for up to one week.

Ginger

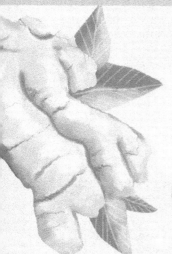

Family:
Zingiberaceae – Ginger Family

Botanical Name:
Zingiber officinale

Other Common Names:
Ginger Root, Common Ginger

Common ginger is a perennial plant that grows annual pseudostems of about three to four feet (90–120 cm) tall. It has been used for many thousands of years as a flavoring and a medicinal. Ginger comes from the same family as turmeric, galangal, and cardamom. We call it ginger root but the part we generally use is really a rhizome (stem).

Native to southeastern Asia, but likely domesticated about 5000 BCE by prehistoric peoples known as Austronesians, ginger was carried all over the world very early in human history. It was known to the ancient Greeks and Romans and was one of the first spices in the spice trade from the orient to Europe.

Ginger is a tropical herb that prefers rich, moist soil, filtered light, and warm, humid weather. It does not tolerate full sun, poor drainage, strong winds, or cold temperatures, and is only hardy in zones 9 –12. Ginger clumps need to be about two years old before they flower. The flowers develop in groups on their own stems, directly from the rhizome, and form white and pink buds that open to reveal flowers with yellow petals that have purple edges. They are little but colorful.

Propagation

Ginger is grown from pieces of rhizome saved from a previous crop. Untreated rhizomes, purchased at a natural foods store, can give you a start. Choose a rhizome that is plump and healthy looking, not shriveled at all. Each piece must have at least one bud from which the first stems will come. Plant your pieces about three inches (7 cm) deep, with the bud upwards, one or two to a twelve inch (30 cm) pot. If planting in the ground, place about eight inches (20 cm) apart. Keep the soil moist but not soggy; mulch thickly to reduce watering and add organic matter.

Ginger is a pot plant in colder climates as it takes a minimum of ten months to grow mature rhizomes to harvest. A pot allows your herb to spend the summer outside and then come in when the nights start to get cool. For **Maintenance** Keep ginger well weeded, It doesn't like competition from other plants. When your ginger starts to die back, reduce watering and allow the soil to dry out.

Spider mites can be a problem in dry air, especially when ginger is grown indoors. Misting with water can help. Poorly drained soil contributes to root rot. Leaf spot and fusarium wilt can sometimes be an issue as well.

My entire life, I have had serious issues with motion sickness. That is especially upsetting because I live near some absolutely gorgeous mountains but cannot enjoy driving through them. My mom loved to drive through the mountain scenery in the fall, taking in the changing colors of the leaves. My husband enjoys the same drives and I am unable to join in at all, without help. Unfortunately, that trait has been passed down to my children. Thankfully, ginger is a champion at calming the nausea and vomiting of motion/sea sickness, pregnancy, illness, and cancer treatment.

Ginger also reduces the gas and bloating of an upset stomach and it has strong anti-inflammatory properties that relieve the pain of menstrual cramps, sore muscles and aching joints. Ginger also has immune-boosting and antiviral constituents that provide relief when ill, clearing sinuses, congestion and sore throats. It improves circulation and is often taken with other herbs to assist in assimilating them. New research shows that it may also be useful in reducing the fasting blood sugar levels in diabetics. As far as **Safety** goes, it's GRAS, but higher doses (0.2 oz – five grams – or more) may cause burping and heartburn in some people.

Ginger is used as a spice, particularly popular in Asian dishes. It is dried and ground to add flavor to seafood, meats, rice, curries, vegetable casseroles, ice cream, and other desserts such as cookies and cakes. It is the main flavoring in ginger snaps and gingerbread. Young rhizomes are fleshy, mild and often eaten as a vegetable or pickled in vinegar or wine. Mature, fresh rhizomes flavor candy, or are candied and eaten as a sweetmeat, or are used to flavor teas. Other culinary uses include carbonated drinks such as ginger ale and ginger beer, and alcoholic drinks. Ginger flowers are edible and can be added to salads, used to decorate cakes or placed as a garnish.

Other Uses

The fragrant ginger plant is often used as a landscape flower around tropical homes. The showier flowering gingers are edible, but they just don't taste as good. There is even a variegated cultivar.

Harvest

Small pieces of rhizome can be broken off after about four months. Harvest them without bothering the rest of the rhizome. It takes about ten months to reach maturity. Dig the rhizomes after the stalks wither. Whole ginger rhizome will keep fresh just on the counter (like a potato) for about ten days, or will last in a plastic bag in the refrigerator for several weeks. It can be frozen, candied or cut into small pieces and dried for long-term storage.

4 cups ginger, young, non-fibrous rhizome (root), scraped and cut into ¼ inch (0.6 cm) squares or slices

Water to cover

2 cups sugar, granulated

1 cup light corn syrup

1 lemon, seeded and sliced with peel

Sugar, granulated or a bit bigger (in which to roll the finished ginger)

- Put the ginger in a non-reactive saucepan and cover with water. Bring to a boil, turn down the heat and simmer until the ginger is tender, about 20 minutes.

- Add 1 cup sugar and bring to a boil. Remove from heat, cover, and let stand at room temperature for four hours to overnight.

- Add the lemon slices and corn syrup. Reheat to a boil, and simmer for 15 minutes more.
  Again, remove from heat and let stand 4 hours to overnight.

- Add 1 cup sugar. Reheat to a boil and again simmer for 30 minutes more. During this third reheating, stir often to prevent scorching. Again, let it stand for four hours to overnight.

- Add 1 cup sugar. Bring to a boil and simmer, stirring frequently. When the syrup drops heavily from the side of the spoon and the ginger is translucent, it's done.

- At this point you can either pour the ginger pieces and syrup into small canning jars and seal, or drain and let the ginger dry overnight on a cooling rack. Reserve the ginger syrup to use in tea or to flavor other dishes.

- When the candied ginger is well dried, roll in granulated or decorative sugar. Store between wax paper in a tin, in a cool, dry place until needed.

32 More Herbs to Grow as You Master Herbalism

Congratulations! You got this far and learned about 21 herbs! I wanted to make this book more affordable for you so I decided to cut the printing costs by providing a PDF file containing details on 32 more herbs for you to learn about, grow and use.

You can get it in a few clicks or by scanning the QR code below. I want you to get more BANG for your buck. This book was made with love for you, our future herbalist. Enjoy!

https://theherb.space/32herbs/

Planting and Propagating Your Herbs

How to Grow From Cuttings

Root and Rhizome Cuttings

Nana taught me that one way to propagate existing perennial plants and still have the same cultivar as the original plant, is to use a root cutting. It is a method unfamiliar to many gardeners but isn't hard to do. The method is not appropriate for every plant. Check under the propagation details for specific species to determine if this method is appropriate for your herb.

1. A piece of root is taken in the late fall or the spring but usually before the herb breaks dormancy. Roots have a high level of energy before they start their spring growth so a root cutting at that time is more likely to be successful. The roots used should be firm and white, at least as thick as a pencil lead and at least two inches (5 cm) in length. Examine carefully and discard any roots with insect or disease damage.

2. Dip the cuttings in rooting hormone. Commercial rooting hormone is a synthetic version of auxin, a hormone that plants naturally make to grow roots, and is usually sold as a powder in small jars. It may be found at most garden centers and greenhouses where you can purchase plants. There is usually enough moisture in a root that when you dip it in, the root comes out white. The hormone allows your success rate to increase, from rooting six out of ten cuttings to nine out of ten. Only herbs that are easy to root, like pineapple sage or pussy willow, have ten out of ten statistics.

3. Place cuttings into a moist, sterile rooting mix. Make sure to position each cutting top side up; the top is usually thicker than the root lower down.

4. Cover loosely with about half an inch of mix and keep damp but not wet. Depending on the specific herb, new growth should show above the soil in two to six weeks.

5. When the growth shows, remove the cover, provide light, and feed like you would any house plant.

6. The herbs can be planted outside, if desired, when big enough and weather allows.

Rhizomes are slightly different from roots, botanically, but they are used in a similar way for propagation. The biggest difference is that you must make sure every piece of rhizome you select for propagation has a bud from which the new growth will appear.

Dipping roots and rhizomes in rooting hormones will get the cuttings off to a healthy start and increase the chances of success. Make your own rooting hormone from apple cider vinegar. A teaspoon of vinegar in 5 to 6 cups (1.2–1.5 liters) of water is enough. The type of apple cider vinegar at your local supermarket is fine. Resist the temptation to use a greater amount, as too much will actually kill your herb. Straight vinegar is used to kill weeds in driveways, walks and other places where plant growth is unwanted. I know many who swear by using cinnamon in the place of rooting hormone as well.

Stem Cuttings

Many herbs will grow from stem cuttings and making them is a fairly easy way to increase your herbs while ensuring the new baby has the same properties or is the same cultivar as the parent herb.

1. Cut a 6–8 inch (15–20 cm) section of each stem. Ensure that the length you cut has at least two to four leaf nodes present; one or two will be planted below ground and the others will be above the surface. Water the parent plant a day to several hours before taking the cuttings to make sure that these will be full of water. The cuttings won't be able to take up water until new roots grow.

2. Remove leaves from the part of the stem that will be below ground.

3. Dip the bottom half of the cutting in rooting hormone, if using; it isn't essential for easy to root plants but increases your success. Pot up your cuttings. Place the stem covered with the hormone below the soil, and the leafy part above ground. You can put each cutting in its own little pot or around the edge of a larger pot. A six inch (15 cm) pot will hold eight to ten cuttings without crowding. The soil should be light, sterile, and moist but not soggy.

4. Pinch out the growing tip leaving just two or four leaves above ground. That serves two purposes: the first is to reduce water loss through the leaves, and the second is to enable you to identify new growth that will prove your cuttings have grown roots.

5. If the air is dry, a clear plastic bag can be placed over each pot to increase the humidity; this will decrease water loss.

6. Some plants grow roots faster than others. You should see new growth in 4–8 weeks.

7. Refrain from adding fertilizer until

you are sure the herb has rooted. Then use half-strength organic fertilizer, compost tea or nettle tea.

A variation of this is to pull off a small branch (not cut off) leaving a bit of the heel attached. I've used this method on woody stems such as elder and rosemary. Otherwise the rest of the directions are the same. Roots grow from this tissue sooner than from the leaf nodes, which speeds up the process.

Some herbs with soft stems will root in a glass of water. It has been successful for me with herbs such as basil. One year, I had basil propagating everywhere and used those baby plants to gift to family and friends. Some consider this method not to be a good idea because roots that 'breathe' under water are very different from roots that 'breathe' in soil. I don't personally use this method very often but if you choose to, you should keep an eye on the roots and transfer the cutting into soil as soon as the roots appear. Definitely do this by the time the roots are an eighth of an inch (3 mm) long. It is easy to lose cuttings if you allow the roots to grow too long.

Layering

This is a method for hard-to-root herbs including woody ones, like thyme and winter savory. Since the stem is still fed by the parent herb, the time it takes for the cutting to root doesn't affect success.

1. Choose a young stem or branch you can bend down to the ground. The stem should be a year old or younger.

2. Leaving the stem attached, bend it down until it touches the ground.

3. Scrape the outer bark off the underside where the stem touches the soil, and peg it down. Hair pins, opened paper clips, or just short wires bent into a 'U' shape are good for this. You can also use a brick or rock to hold the stem down.

4. After pegging, cover the stem with potting soil or compost. Water to settle and moisten the soil.

5. Pinch out the growing tip.

6. Keep the soil moist but not wet.

7. In four to eight weeks you should see new growth on most plants. New growth shows that roots have developed. Know the specifics about your plant; some species can take up to two years to root in this way.

8. Once rooted, cut the stem from the parent plant and pot up or plant the new herb as a transplant.

Dividing Perennials

My children always look forward to the time of year when we divide our plants. We make it a family affair and we all get a little section to add to our personal gardens. We do this because I feel like it's important to teach the love of gardening and herbalism to my children as well. You can also make more of a good thing by dividing your herbs that clump, every three to four years. Dividing also reinvigorates perennial herbs that become crowded when they get overgrown. Some of these include chives, purple coneflower and most of the mint family. An exception is lavender.

1. The best time of year to divide perennials is late spring or early fall. You know your local weather best and plants recover better in the cool (not cold) and rainy weather of those seasons. If do divide an herb in mid-summer, check it often and water it to keep the summer heat from drying out the roots.

2. Water the area several days before dividing. This will soften the soil and make digging less work. It also ensures the plant has taken up all the water it can hold; it will need this until it can recover from having its roots disturbed.

3. Dig up the clump you wish to divide. Insert the shovel all the way around the clump. Using the shovel under the root ball, lift it as a single piece.

4. After it's out of the ground, shake or brush loose dirt away so you can see the root ball and decide where to divide.

5. Using your shovel or a sharp knife, cut apart the individual growing crowns in the clump. Make sure each smaller clump has at least one set of leaves attached to roots.

6. Add a shovelful of compost to the soil for each new clump. This improves the moisture-holding capacity of your soil plus adds the nutrients that the new perennials will need.

7. Replant the new clumps at the same depth they sat originally and with the recommended spacing in between. It will look like a lot of space at first but the plants will need that space as they grow.

8. Keep the soil moist but not soggy until the herb recovers from being divided, which should take about four weeks.

Growing From Seed

How to Choose the Right Seeds for Your Garden

One way I cope with winter is to pour over my many seed catalogs. I circle and highlight and dream of all the seeds I want to plant in my garden and yard. How do you decide what to grow? It can be tempting to buy one of every type (remember, you can't possibly weed THAT many), but there can be a method to the seed-buying madness.

First, make a general list. What would you like to grow? Ask yourself honestly, "Will my family really eat/use that?" Yes, it's healthy and you *should* eat that (for example, holy basil or kale), but there is no sense in spending your hard-earned cash on seed, and your all-too-short spare time on weeding something, when you know deep down they will not eat it. Do you want mainly a culinary herb garden? A medicinal one? Do you make your own cosmetics? Personally, I adore going outside to my garden knowing that I have all these options in mine, mostly in the form of multi-purpose plants like mint, oregano, rosemary, lavender, sage, and calendula.

Secondly, identify the needs of the plants you wish to grow. Do they need sun or will they tolerate shade? As much as I'd like to, there are some things I just can't grow where I live. Also how big is your garden area? How many of your chosen plants can you fit into the allotted space? Crowded plants get disease more easily and may not perform well. Being realistic will save you time, money and frustration!

Make lists. Pick the specific varieties of the things you wish to grow. Plants have been bred for many different traits. For example, thyme: there are tall ones, creeping ones, variegated ones and ones with different flavors. Pick those that are perfect for your needs. I make lists of things I want to try, and then edit and re-edit the list until I get down to a manageable number. If I ever win the lottery, I am going to hire a full-time gardener to weed all the things I'd like to plant!

Buy your seeds. At first glance it may seem like all seed companies are alike but this is most definitely not the case.

Local garden centers can be a good choice, especially for beginners, because trained staff can answer your questions. Also there is something to be said for instant gratification; I love walking in to browse and walking out clutching my choices. However,

there is a greater choice offered in seed catalogs (physical books as well as online options) and many provide information about cultivation to improve your chances of success. While most gardening catalogs carry some herbs, there are specialty catalogs just for herbs and these have a bigger selection. Seed catalogs are usually sent out starting in late November and many advertise financial incentives to order before February, but you can order most of the different types throughout the year. Some seeds are so popular that they may run out before spring.

Whichever source you use and whatever seeds you choose, keep a written record of the varieties you plant and evaluate them as they grow. Use this knowledge to assist in purchasing the following year.

Light Requirements

Most commonly grown herbs are sun lovers that prefer six to eight hours of full sunlight each day. Some grow best in shade. Those plants will grow fine when started under artificial light, but later will need protection from the strong light in a greenhouse. Seeds started outside are best grown in their permanent home.

How Deep Should I Plant My Seeds?

Burying seed too deep will affect germination. Herb babies will have to struggle up to the light and may not make it if they have too far to go. Many seeds require light to trigger germination and stay dormant when planted too deep. Buried in the ground, some last for many years until the soil is disturbed, thus bringing them up to the

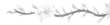

light. These are often the tiny seeds. A rule of thumb is to plant seeds no deeper than they are big. Very fine seed is best just pressed into the surface of the soil.

Domestic seed has been bred to germinate all at the same time after planting. Herbs that are more wild have not. Wild seed often has what is referred to as delayed germination. Only some of the seed comes up in the first growing season, some in the second, and more in the third. If the spring is too wet and the baby plants suffer root rot, or drought affects the area and the seedlings wilt and die, there are more seeds to ensure the survival of the species.

How to Stratify Seeds

Some herbs need to be stratified to trigger germination, while others sprout better if stratified. That is a fancy term for going through a cold spell that mimics the winter season with its low temperatures. You control the time of sprouting when you artificially stratify the seed. Using your refrigerator to stratify also avoids those out-of-season warm spells that climate change has caused in some places. Those warm spells can last long enough to fool herbs into breaking dormancy and sprouting early, only to die when the weather turns cold again. Young seedlings are much more susceptible to cold temperatures. Since seed is not cheap, you want most to thrive. If you're lucky, you'll get eight out of ten seeds to sprout and if you're very lucky, you'll get ten out of ten.

To start plants inside before the weather stabilizes, place seed overnight in a handful of damp, sterile soil in a small, recycled clam shell container with a clear top, or in a ziplock bag. Planting in peat pellets also works well. Label and date each variety clearly. Then place in a refrigerator for between one and three months. Specific information is given in the details about each herb in this book. With purchased seed the instructions are usually provided on each seed packet. Check at least once and water if necessary, to keep the soil damp but not soggy. A plant mister helps add water without overwatering.

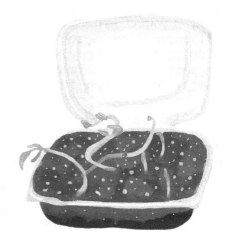

After the stratification period has passed, plant the seeds as usual in flats or pots and place in a warm, well-lit location. You can skip the planting if the seed is already in peat pots or cell packs.

How to Sow Seeds in Winter

If stratification seems like too much work, or your family objects to several clam shells full of dirt in your refrigerator, plant your seed in place, just as you would when it's warm outside. In cold areas it's also possible to sprinkle your seeds in place over the snow; they will drop down to the soil as the snow melts and provides the moisture needed for the seeds to germinate as spring comes and the soil warms.

But hungry birds and small rodents may be an issue if you use this method.

Growing From a Young Plant

I am absolutely terrible about walking through the garden center at the store, going to a plant nursery, or my local Mennonite farm looking at transplants. I often have to talk myself out of buying a lot of young transplants and focus instead on starting from seeds. I'm impatient sometimes (as I'm sure we all can be) and starting things from seeds can take a while, and require space that I sometimes just don't have.

Whether started from seeds, cuttings or division, transplants are a convenient way to plant your herb garden. Starting seeds early lets you get a head start on the summer season. Purchased transplants, on the other hand, allow you to get a head start when you don't have the room or the light to start plants indoors. For other herbs, it's the only way to ensure you buy a specific cultivar.

You are paying for another person's time and labor so transplants are not cheap. Last summer they started at $4.50 each, for easy-to-start herbs, and went up in price from there. We've been told to expect a higher price next summer. If you only need one or two individuals of some particular herb, it may be better to buy transplants than to be stuck with seeds you won't use. If you plan to buy one to get

hold of a specific cultivar, make sure to propagate it yourself afterwards. Hybrids don't breed true, their seed reverts to the characteristics of one parent or the other or, worse still, may be sterile and fail to germinate at all.

Or if you win the lottery, you may want to purchase loads of transplants to give yourself an instant garden.

Since transplanting is hard on plants, be sure your seedlings are ready to face the cold, cruel world. The herbs should have at least two pairs of true leaves, be at least three inches (7.5 cm) high, and be properly hardened off.

Similar to tanning at home so you won't burn when vacationing at the beach, hardening off means slowly getting a plant used to the sun and wind outside. They are used to the lack of wind and to the low light conditions of indoor growing. The strongest light of an indoor setup is nothing like the strength of direct sunlight. Only expensive grow lamps or a greenhouse come close.

Put your seedlings in a protected place outside for two hours then put them back inside in their usual place. Do it again the next day. The third day, take them out for four hours. Repeat, the next day. On the fifth day, leave the plants outside for six hours and repeat that the following day. By the seventh day, the chlorophyll in your transplant's leaves will have built up and your herbs will be ready to stay out all day. They are now ready to be planted outside.

A. The morning of the big day, or at least two hours before the event, water your plants.

B. Dig a hole twice the size of the herb you plan to put in it.

C. Mix a handful of compost into the dirt at the bottom of the hole.

D. Carefully un-pot the seedling. If it was started in a peat pellet, peat pot or soil block, plant the whole thing as it is. You may need to tear off some of the peat pot to plant the whole thing. If you leave some of the peat pot above the soil, it will act like a wick and will dry out the pot.

If the transplant has grown too large, it may be pot-bound. That is a term that means the dirt is completely full of roots and they've grown around each other. Most herbs in this condition benefit from having their roots unwound. This is also a reason not to buy plants that are already blooming: they'll be stunted and pot-bound. Perennials usually recover eventually, but annuals rarely do. But not all plants like to have their roots unwound. If the herb is a member of the Apiaceae family (for example, parsley, dill, coriander) and was started in a conventional cell pack or pot, be careful! These herbs hate to have their roots disturbed but can be planted from a start if they're small and you're careful to not break their tap root. Your herb will be stunted if you do, and may die. These same plants can't be dug up and moved once established.

1. Plant your new transplants at the same level as the herb grew before. True mints will grow roots along a buried stem, but most other herbs don't do well if they are planted deeper.

2. Pat down, then water to settle the dirt.

3. Keep the new transplants damp, but not wet, until the herb becomes established. That will take about two weeks.

Harvesting and Storing Your Herbs

I have always loved gardening. But my first year of having my very own herb garden was something really special because it was the first time I could harvest something that had grown solely due to my own hard work and efforts. I used a wooden basket and carefully cut sprigs of various herbs. The aroma that wafted from my basket every time it moved was positively intoxicating.

When is The Best Time to Harvest?

Flowers are at their best when first open. Pick them daily to avoid self-sowing. Some seeds are toxic, and all of them take a lot of energy from the plant while they are forming. Only allow seeds to ripen if you have annuals or want to increase your plants by means of seeds. I also leave some flowers for the pollinators and only harvest them at the very last minute.

Harvest most **leaves** at their strongest, when the flavor is best and the medicinal constituents most powerful. The general rule is to cut leaves when flower buds have formed but not yet opened , or when just a few blooms on the spike have opened. Much strength is expended by the plant in flowering and ripening seed. Some herbs are strong enough to be used any time that they're big enough, but they will be stronger still at the proper time. Exceptions to this rule are covered in the information about specific herbs.

Rhizomes are modified stems that grow underground. A rhizome grows horizontally with shoots growing upwards from buds and roots sprouting off and growing downwards. They store plant nutrients and allow the herb to spread laterally. Harvest rhizomes in the autumn, just like roots.

Roots may be harvested from fall to early spring, when the plant has sent all its goodies down to be stored for dormant season and they have not yet been used in breaking dormancy.

The best time to harvest the roots of annuals and any other roots destined for the cook pot is early in the first autumn. At this time, the roots haven't sustained any grub or rodent damage that might occur during the winter, and they are still tender. Most roots become woody when sending up flower stalks. The first autumn is also the best time to harvest roots of biennials as they are usually dead by the second fall.

You may wish to wait for perennials to get strong and spread a bit before harvesting any of their roots. In that case the second or even the third autumn is better. Roots meant for food are more tender the first fall but perennial roots meant as medicine are better harvested the second autumn. Most perennial plants stay small during the first growing season and you don't want to endanger the survival of your perennials by gathering before there is enough root left behind for the plant.

Harvesting from The Wild

Wild crafting can be very satisfying. Be very sure that you have identified the plant correctly, however, before using any part of it. Don't use herbs from roadsides where the soil may be contaminated by chemicals and automobile exhaust. It hasn't been that long since we added lead to gasoline. Lead and herbicides used to control weeds along roadways are usually found in the top few inches of soil and persist for many years. Mullein is an example of an herb that is of great medicinal value but is often found in the wild near roadsides. This has been my very unhappy experience, anyway. How frustrating

it is finding something so useful yet being unable to harvest any of it!

You can gather seeds from herbs that you find, and grow them in your garden or in a guerilla garden, thus ensuring the resulting herbs are safe to use. Make sure any seed gathered from plants in the wild is fully ripe or it won't germinate.

Storing Your Herbs

Light and moisture degrade the flavor and medical constituents of herbal products; ultimately, these factors can also destroy the physical condition of your herbs and herbal products as well. Whether in short- or long-term storage, herbs and herbal products keep best in a cool, dry, dark location. If the only place you have to store them is well lit, cover the storage jars or use amber and blue containers that filter out much of the light. You can cover the jars with fancy blackboard paint or cost-effective paper; they both do the job. Sunlight is the biggest issue but artificial light exposure should be kept minimal as well.

Dried herbs keep longer in whole or large pieces as there is less surface area exposed to the air. Crush or powder them as needed.

Short-term Storage

Most dried leaves and flowers will last at least from one harvest to the next. Many will last several years and still be useful for cooking but will require larger amounts as the flavor fades. This is a general rule with exceptions (I'm thinking of lobelia and St. John's wort here) so you must still research each herb. If you keep a notebook, you'll only have to do the research once. Acetums and syrups follow the harvest to harvest rule. Seeds, barks and medicinal roots, because they're encased in fibrous or tough, woody cellulose, will keep for several years once dried.

Long-term Storage

Candied roots, seeds, or berries keep for at least 4 years before losing their flavor. Tinctures and extracts last four to six years for medicinal purposes, and longer if used for flavoring purposes. They will keep for even longer but their properties will diminish. Glycerites keep for two years, as a general rule. Freezing is an option that will preserve herbs for up to two years, if they are well packaged to prevent freezer burn.

Becoming the Guardian Angel of Your Garden

Feeding

Fertilizing

Feeding herbs requires judgment on your part. If your soil test shows poor fertility, follow the recommendations for the first fertilizing. Use organic sources, since the long-range plan is to eat these products. Later, during the growing season, if your herbs look tired or lose their color, you can add fish emulsion or liquid seaweed but the best is to top dress with compost.

Most herbs are not heavy feeders; exceptions are noted under the entry for specific herbs. A high concentration of fertilizer can burn your herbs. Also, the addition of too many nutrients, especially nitrogen, can produce rapid new growth that is soft and very susceptible to disease. Slow release fertilizer is best for the steady growth that you want. A gardener's job requires balance – too much fertilizer is bad, but not enough produces stunted, unhappy herbs. Like the fairy tale, you want things to be just right! I saw this first-hand over the past couple years. Last year, I used fertilizer regularly, mixed in when I watered my plants. They all did wonderfully and produced a lot. This year, I did not use fertilizer regularly and, as a result, my plants weren't as beautiful; but they tasted better and were obviously stronger.
Lesson learned for me.

Making Compost

When we got our chickens at the beginning of the year, it was my first go at keeping them so I read up on them as much as possible. Apart from the obvious advantages of having chickens (eggs and meat), their waste makes a wonderful addition to our compost! This includes all the stuff I shovel from their run such as the used straw, scraps, and poop all mixed together. Totally gross sounding but amazingly beneficial!

Making compost involves being somewhat like a mad scientist. A bit of this and a bit of that, all mixed up in a pile, and after a while you have black gold. Compost is the very best fertilizer . It improves your soil when added to the original bed or to a pot, or when used as compost tea to water your plants. Although it is theoretically possible, you really have to work hard to have too much. Composting will reduce the amount of waste and kitchen scraps sent to the landfill. Some of the bigger cities have a composting service where you can drop off a full compost bucket and pick up an empty one.

However, if you have the space and get as addicted to gardening as I have, sooner or later you'll make your own. Making your own compost is easy once you understand the process. Most of the work is done by aerobic (oxygen loving) bacteria. There's a method to the mixing and I'm going to explain that here, but first I'm going to cover some basics.

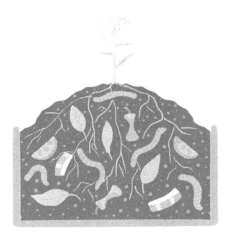

Brown Matter is mostly cellulose. It can be sourced from the following substances:

1. Straw. Don't use hay in a cold pile as there are usually many weed

seeds in it. A hot pile usually kills the weed seeds.

2. Shredded newspaper. This is a perfect use for my paper shredder.

3. Paper bags, shipping boxes, packing paper, shirt board, and other cardboard cut into strips.

4. Autumn leaves.

5. Sawdust or wood chips from untreated wood.

Green Matter contains nitrogen to feed healthy levels of bacteria. For this you can add the following:

1. Grass clippings. Be sure no herbicide was sprayed on them before they were cut

2. Yard waste

3. Coffee grounds

4. Egg shells, vegetable peels, moldy bread and other kitchen waste. Don't add any bones, dairy, meat scraps or fat. These will smell bad as they rot and will attract flies, wasps, and animal pests. Don't include cat or dog feces as this smells bad and may spread some diseases and parasites to humans.. On the other hand, chicken, rabbit, cow, and horse manure can be included as it all makes great fertilizer.

There are two kinds of compost piles. The first is called a **cold pile**. The green and brown matter is layered and left to decay. You can layer leaves with green matter in a trash bag, dampen if necessary, and then tie it closed. Use the sealed bag to insulate a foundation, porch or crawl space; the following spring or summer you can open the bag and use the contents as compost. A cold pile can take nine to twelve months to decay, with smaller pieces taking less time than bigger ones.

The second is called a **hot pile**. A hot pile involves more work than a cold pile, but it decays much faster. The warmth of the summer will mean that, if you use small pieces to begin with and turn the pile regularly, you can have finished compost in a month! I don't know about you but I feel doing a little more work while saving a lot of time is absolutely worth it.

1. Your first step here is to layer the brown and green matter into a large pile in the proportion of three parts brown matter to one part green. Be careful not to add diseased plants or those containing weed seeds to the mix, especially if it isn't going to get hot enough to kill things. You certainly don't want the diseases to spread to your plants when you use the compost. The pile may be simply placed on the ground or it could be in a fancy compost bin. A pile that heats up even in the winter will need to be about three feet (90 cm) high.

2. If your pile doesn't touch the earth (such as in concrete areas, apartments, composting barrels), add a shovelful of finished compost or purchased compost starter to introduce the proper bacteria to your pile. Even if it does touch the earth, you may wish to add bacteria to your first pile in the same way, to speed things up. Afterwards, add a shovelful of your own finished compost to the next pile or build it in the same place to take advantage of the bacteria already in the dirt.

3. Water well to dampen all ingredients and cover the pile with a tarp or plastic drop cloth.

4. Check your pile every week and sprinkle it with water if it doesn't rain. You want the pile to be moist but not soggy. The bacteria that break down the goodies in the pile are aerobic, meaning they need oxygen. A soggy pile will encourage anaerobic bacteria that will make it sour and smelly. Add more brown matter to fix a sour blend. If the mix is too dry the bacteria will stop working and no decay will take place. Dampen it to start things working again.

5. If you want to check the temperature inside the pile you can use a compost thermometer, obtainable from garden supply stores and online catalogs. Or you can just push your hand into the middle of your pile. It should feel warm.

6. Turn your hot pile once a week during the summer months or when the thermometer reads between 130 and 150°F (between 55 and 65°C). It may take a bit longer when it's cold out but a well made pile gets hot enough to steam

even when covered with snow. Turning allows oxygen in, mixes up ingredients to prevent matting, and moves undigested materials into the middle of the pile. It will heat up fast after turning.

7. A compost barrel makes the turning easy; just give it a couple of spins weekly. But it does limit the volume of your production. Compost barrels work well for small gardens and will fit on an apartment balcony. You can even repurpose a 55 gallon (200 liter) drum into a compost barrel!

8. So how do you know when it's done? That one's simple enough. When the ingredients have broken down and the compost no longer gets hot, it's good to go. It should be brown and crumbly and ready for use. I like to have several piles going at once. One building, one or more working and one or more ready to use.

A variation on the cold pile concept is **lasagna gardening**. It's a good way to start a new garden. In the fall, mow the grass very short where you desire the garden to be. Cover the area of the actual garden with cardboard or newsprint five sheets thick. Then add your green and brown matter in alternating layers and allow it time to do its thing. You are basically building a long, low compost pile. By spring, the grass is dead, everything has broken down, and you can plant or transplant directly into the newly formed organic soil.

A way to improve an existing garden is to dig a trench or a hole in a path or unused area. Fill the trench or hole with alternating layers of green and brown matter, as you collect it. It's a great place to empty your kitchen compost pot. Cover the last few inches with the original dirt. Then move over and start to fill the next trench or hole. If your ground freezes hard in the winter, you can dig several trenches or holes ahead of time. They'll be filled by spring. Cover the removed dirt with a tarp or plastic drop cloth until you need it. The level of dirt in the holes will dip down as the ingredients rot; just fill the gaps back to level.

Watering

Manual Watering

My mom always taught me that the best time to water your plants is in the morning. This way the water actually gets down into the soil instead of just evaporating from the surface like it would if watered during the warmth of the day. It is best to water the dirt, not the plants themselves. Watering from the top, like you do when using a sprinkler, gets the leaves wet and encourages the spread and growth of diseases. If you water before dark then the soil and plants don't have time to dry before night falls and this also encourages diseases. But this is the second best time for watering, as long as you wet the soil and not the plants.

If watering pots, indoors or out, water from the bottom. Fill the pot's saucer full of water and let the container stand in it to absorb what the dirt needs. After about an hour, empty the saucer and allow the pot to drain. Do not leave saucers under outside pots;

they'll collect rain and encourage rot.

When using a watering can, again, water the soil not the plants. The same when using a hose; just lay the pipe between plants and allow the water to run for a while, then move it about four feet over and repeat. Below are some alternative methods. If you do choose to use an overhead sprinkler (they are cheap), water in the morning so the plants dry completely before dark.

Leaky Hose (Soaker Hose)

Leaky hose has microscopic holes to allow water to ooze out of the length of the hose. It can be used alone but is usually part of a watering system. The hose should be covered with mulch to prevent sun damage and make the hose last at least several seasons.

Automatic Watering Systems

These are so helpful! They work on a timer, turning on and off at precise times. This means you don't have to be there to water your garden. They are nice when added to a watering system. They take a bit of thought and an investment, but can save you a lot of work and are nice if your time is short during your mornings.

Harvesting Rainwater

This is outlawed in some areas; ignore the following if that's true for your area. I don't encourage anyone to break the law. For other areas, this is a great way to avoid city water which may be harmful to your garden. After all, chemicals are added to city water to prevent algae and other

things from growing in the pipes that carry the water to your home.

One of the easiest ways to collect the rain is to use your roof as a collector and run a downspout into a barrel. You can make a series of barrels, connected together with plastic pipe, and at graduated heights so that when one is full, the overflow fills the others. You can install a tap connection with a cut-off valve in the lowest barrel, to use for watering the garden. Very convenient!

Identifying and Managing Plant Diseases

The best way to deal with problems in the garden is to avoid them in the first place. Easier said than done, I know. But there are effective ways of prevention. The first requirement is to keep a clean garden. Most problems arise when a garden is crowded and messy. All debris, including empty pots, should be removed.

The plants that die from diseases should be put in the trash, not on the compost pile. Fact of the matter is, we just can't be sure the whole pile will get hot enough to kill all the viruses, fungi and bacteria. Compost is supposed to do the garden good, not spread disease.

When you plant your seeds or transplants, make sure they are placed the recommended distance apart for good air circulation. They'll never do well if they can't 'breathe' properly.

Keep your herbs healthy by giving each

plant what it needs. Insects and diseases tend to bother unhealthy plants. I make this easier on myself by planting things with similar needs together.

Water the soil, not the leaves. Overhead watering spreads many diseases. If you can, water in the morning so plants and soil surface have time to dry before dark.

If you've done everything you can to avoid problems and suffer one anyway, the most common problems are listed below, along with the best organic treatments.

Aphids

Aphids, in addition to the damage they do themselves, leave behind a sticky liquid called 'honeydew.' This honeydew grows mold and viruses. Sometimes the aphids are farmed and 'milked' for this fluid by ants. Ants themselves usually don't pose any sort of threat but getting rid of the ants helps keep aphid populations down since ants protect the aphids from predators such as lacewings or ladybugs that hunt them down and eat them. Trim the bottom leaves and coat the stem with something sticky so the ants cannot climb up. Most aphids

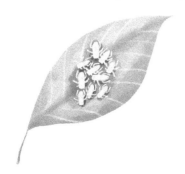

wash off with a spray of water but sometimes you need a stronger control.

You can actually buy ladybugs and lacewings so you may want to give them a try first. Even organic pesticides will kill good bugs with the bad. As a last resort, use insecticidal soap or neem oil. Be sure to wash herbs well before using. Diatomaceous earth is also another natural option that is plant safe but deadly for aphids and many other insects. Wear a mask when applying this. Breathing in DE dust will cut the delicate tissue inside your lungs resulting in scar tissue.

Bacterial Leaf spot

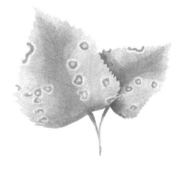

There isn't any known cure for this bacterial disease so control is important. This problem first shows up, and is more common, on older leaves and then moves to newer growth. The bacteria that cause it favor cool, rainy conditions. It can overwinter on herb debris and seeds, and then splash up from there. Choose resistant cultivars when available, pick disease-free transplants, and avoid overhead watering. For serious infections, solarize the soil and don't grow any susceptible herbs the following season.

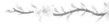

Black Spot Fungus

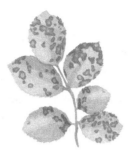

Even though it commonly affects roses, it also affects other herbs. Inspect your herbs often so you catch any signs of black spot fungus early. Ten minutes of scrutiny every morning is better than spending two hours checking up each weekend. I stroll through my garden with my cup of tea, pulling this and picking that, every morning before work. It catches problems early and allows me to make plans for later harvests. I also find it very relaxing to be in my garden before the day really starts. If you can't manage a morning trip, take a walk in the evening and destress while you care for your garden.

The fungus starts growing when the temperature reaches 60°F (16°C) and the garden has been wet for six to nine hours – perfect rainy, spring weather. Temperatures over 85°F (30°C) cause the fungus to slow down.

A good general organic antifungal spray can be made by dissolving 4 teaspoons of potassium bicarbonate in 1 gallon (about 4 liters) of water. Baking soda is **sodium** bicarbonate and can be used in an emergency, but potassium bicarbonate really works better. Add a tablespoon of cooking oil and a tablespoon of soap (real soap, not detergent) as well. Pyrethrin leaves

and neem oil are organic controls but will kill the good bugs with the bad. They are safe for all warm-blooded animals such as dogs, cats and rabbits. Keep both away from fish, lizards and insects, though.

Or make your own Bordeaux mixture, a traditional copper-based garden fungicide.

Fire Blight

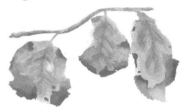

This disease is caused by a bacterium called *Erwinia amylovora*, which affects many plants, shrubs and trees. Fire blight gets its name from the burnt look of affected stems and twigs. The bacteria are spread in splashes of water (rain, overhead watering), on gardening tools, and by insects and birds. Unfortunately, there is no cure, chemical or organic. The best organic remedies are avoiding overhead watering, mulching to prevent splashing, and regular removal of infected plants or branches.

A variety of inorganic sprays can be used to control fire blight. Most of them contain fixed copper.

Remember this is to control, not treat. Control requires a regular schedule of spraying, started in early spring, to impact the bacteria's ability to survive long enough to reproduce and spread. Avoid spreading the bacteria by disinfecting gardening tools, such as pruning shears, used to cut off diseased parts; dip them in straight rubbing alcohol or a chlorine bleach mixture between every cut. Bleach mixture is one part bleach to nine parts water. A part can be a tablespoon or a cup, as long as you use the same measure for each liquid.

Fusarium Wilt

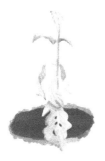

Of all the issues out there, this fungus is probably the most common problem that gardeners face. It affects many herbs and it can live in the soil forever. A common name for it in the greenhouse world is 'the yellows.' The fungus enters the roots of young herbs, blocking the vessels and limiting or completely blocking the plant's ability to transport water and nutrients to its aerial parts. Wilting, that doesn't respond to watering, is usually the first sign of this disease.

Fusarium wilt is associated with warm temperatures and doesn't usually show up outside until days get hot. Remove diseased leaves to slow the spread, and wash off pruners (and any equipment used) between cuts. If this disease occurs inside, sterilize the pots and replace the soil. Remove

all contaminated plant debris and put it in the trash (or burn, if allowed).

Damping Off

This fungus usually affects seedlings in low light, damp and cool conditions. High humidity increases the danger of infection. The fungus rots the plant away at, or just below, the soil surface, causing it to fall over suddenly and die.

The first sign you will see is that your herbs fall over and by then it's usually too late to do anything. There are ways to prevent it, though. Indoors, provide strong light and ensure the soil surface dries out before watering again. Water from the bottom and don't allow water to stay in the saucer, if you use one. Disinfect pots before reuse and discard or heat sterilize contaminated soil. Use sterile soil for starting seedlings indoors for transplant. Outside, water early in the day so plants can dry before dark, make sure your soil drains well, and resort to raised beds if your native soil drains poorly.

Avoidance is best as there is no cure for herbs already affected by damping off. But powdered corn gluten, sprinkled on the surface of the soil, is an organic treatment that has shown promise in controlling soil already contaminated.

Powdery Mildew

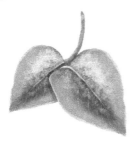

This common fungus is a pain in the rear for most gardeners. It is named for the white powdery covering on most of the leaves, and eventually, the stems and flowers. Some herbs are more susceptible than others. Buy resistant cultivars if available. Plant in full sun if the plant prefers that and encourage good air circulation with adequate spacing. Strong plants are not as susceptible so take all steps to make sure your plants are as healthy as possible. Water the ground to keep leaves dry and mulch to prevent splashing.

You can do everything correctly and still have a problem with this fungus; after all, you can't control the weather. The fungus grows in conditions of high humidity, like in the area where I live. Some days the humidity is so much that it feels like I'm walking through a steam room. Some areas have problems in the warm days and cool nights of early summer, and others in the autumn. Remove dead or diseased foliage.

There are several organic preventions and controls.

1. Spray with one part milk diluted in two parts water. It must be dairy milk and not one of the nut milks. This must come in contact for the milk to work so be sure to spray the underside of leaves. The science behind this is not fully understood but it has been proven not only to deter the fungus but also to boost the plant's immune system.

2. Use the potassium bicarbonate/water/soap mixture described to control black spot fungus.

3. You can also use commercial organic fungicides that list sulfur as an active ingredient.

Root Rot

Lack of oxygen due to prolonged overwatering is the most common cause of root rot. It is easy to keep a plant too wet in a pot that is too big. Outside, heavy clay soil with poor drainage will smother a plant's roots. Take the time to improve the soil in the whole garden area and add compost; and if native soil is really heavy, add sand before planting. Don't improve just the soil in the hole for the plant. All that will do is act like a bucket, holding water and taking a long time to drain.

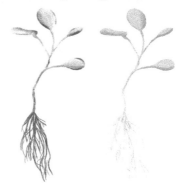

Root rot is also caused by a fungus carried in the soil. When the herb is overwatered once or twice, the dormant spores of this fungus suddenly come to life and infect the roots. Healthy roots are firm and pliable, regardless of color. Dead or dying roots are black and mushy and may fall off when you touch them.

Either situation can be fixed if it's caught early enough. Carefully wash off all the original dirt and remove all dead and decaying roots. If you remove much of the roots, prune back the top growth as well. The herb will not be able to take up water until new roots grow. Dip the remaining healthy roots in fungicide diluted according to the instructions on the label. Repot in a clean, sterile potting mix. It may seem to make sense to fertilize but resist the temptation as this may stress the herb. If the original pot was too large, use a smaller pot of more appropriate size. Hopefully the herb will recover. When you see new growth on top, you'll know the same has happened below. You can replant if you have improved the drainage, or leave the plant in its new pot. Oh, and be sure to dispose of the affected soil.

Scale

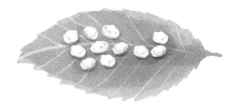

Scale insects are aggravating critters that are small and flat, with a protective shell-like covering (the scale). Scale is usually found on the undersides of leaves and around the stems where leaves attach. There are three kinds of scale insects: armored scale, mealybugs, and soft scale. Scale insects can't fly so they spread by crawling. Removing low leaves and putting sticky tape or goo on the stem will trap crawlers.

Armored scale doesn't make honeydew or white fluffy stuff and is the hardest to get rid of. Insecticidal soap is the best way to get rid of scale especially if you time your application with the emergence of the 'crawlers' from their mothers' shells. Repeat the spraying every six weeks to eventually kill them all.

Mealybugs are easy to identify as they leave a white, cottony residue on the leaves or stems at the leaf nodes. The bugs themselves are small, flat, white spots that suck their nutrition from the herbs. One bug won't hurt your plant but they quickly multiply. If the herb only has a few colonies, a simple fix is to use a cotton-tipped applicator dipped in a mixture of one part alcohol to three parts water. If the infestation is serious, use insecticidal soap.

Soft scale makes a sticky residue called honeydew (yep, the same stuff that aphids make) that provides conditions for the growth of sooty mold, meaning you could have two problems. Ants often care for and spread scale (the same way they do with aphids), feeding on the honeydew produced by these insect pests. Rinse off the honeydew. After drying, spray with insecticidal soap and apply sticky tape or goo to catch the ants.

Slugs and Snails

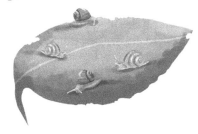

I honestly love slugs and snails. They are fascinating creatures, in my opinion. That being said, they can do much damage to your garden in just one night, munching away at your favorite plants . I have lost many herbs to them. Slugs and snails will eat anything but prefer the tenderness of new growth. They need moisture in order to move about, and leave a mucous trail you can see and follow. They hide from the sun under mulch, boards, rocks, pots, and leaves that are too close together, coming out each evening or when it's overcast. Snakes, toads, chickens and ducks eat them. However, those birds will also eat your seedlings and sometimes, your other plants too so be careful if you decide to use them as biological slug or snail control.

Discourage slugs and snails by putting a circle of crushed eggshells or diatomaceous earth around tender herbs and seedlings. To kill them, one of the best known and most recommended methods I've come across is to put out a pan of beer. Slugs and snails will be attracted and drown in the beer. The downside is that these need to be refreshed or replaced after each rain and it rains often here. A three foot (1 m) piece of smooth board, or an upside down melon rind placed nearby, will attract these pests. Then go out to the garden the next morning to collect and dispose of the slugs or snails that have collected. You keep a jar half filled with salt water to drop them into, throwing the whole thing away every few days. You can also toss the snails and slugs, or the rind, off in the woods or somewhere else if you prefer not to kill them.

Thin plants out to the recommended distance to allow good air circulation to dry things out. Keep the garden area clean, removing rocks, empty pots, and other boards. Raise pots off the ground so slugs can't hide under them. There are cute little feet made to lift big pots, but small pebbles or glass marbles will work as well.

Spider Mites

If you see webs on the tips of your herbs that remind you of the ones spiders make, you probably have this pest. They are a bigger problem in greenhouses or indoors but they do occur on outdoor plants as well. There are many types and they are actually arachnids (closely related to spiders) and not insects. There are the usual predatory insects outside but if they're not doing the job properly you can apply insecticidal soap or neem oil to rid your herbs of these pests.

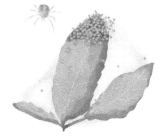

Whiteflies

I've only had this problem indoors, in late winter, when the air is dry and the plants are weak from low light. But I've read that whiteflies can be a real problem in a greenhouse and in warm areas. If you see little white flying things, you probably have whiteflies. Natural predators outdoors include ladybugs, lace wings, and pirate bugs. Keeping your herbs healthy is a good prevention method, but if you have whiteflies on your herbs you can spray them off using water under pressure, thus reducing their numbers. Whiteflies are resistant to most insecticides but neem oil is still effective.

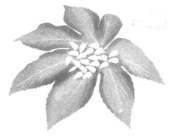

Discouraging the Critters and Wiring Your Containers

Nothing is as discouraging to me as spending lots of time and energy on my garden, only to have local birds, rabbits, squirrels, mice, chipmunks, or deer reap the rewards by chomping off bits just as I'm ready to harvest. They can do much damage in one night.

Blood meal repels with its smell while providing nitrogen. Cayenne pepper works on most rodents and deer. Birds can't taste spice so hot peppers don't work on them.

I have several pieces of hardware cloth bent to have three inch (7.5 cm) sides and a top, to protect seeds from the birds until they get their second leaves. The birds then usually leave them alone.

Tying bars of strong-smelling soap up onto shrubs and trees will deter deer. Deer are creatures of habit, so it's important to put out the soap in the early spring when the deer are setting up their routes. I just put a hole through the middle of the bar and hang it roughly at deer nose level in the area I want to protect. Use a bar every hundred feet or so and check the bars

every couple of weeks to see if they need replacing. The bars last a long time but exactly how long will depend on the amount of rain your area gets.

Fences help with most rodents and, if the fencing mesh is small enough chipmunks and baby rabbits can't go through. Deer can jump a six foot (1.8 m) fence, so you will need a high one if you mean to stop the deer. As a last resort, you can install an electric fence, the height of which will depend on the invaders you're trying to repel.

Weed Control

Solarizing

This can make your gardening experience so much easier. Solarization is an environmentally friendly method of sterilizing the garden using the sun to super heat the soil. It not only kills or weakens diseases in contaminated soil, but also weed seeds for many inches down. It is used in gardens, organic farms and other places where chemical controls are not wanted. It's perfect for herbs! If the surface temperature reaches 140°F (60°C) the soil below, to a depth of about 12 inches (30 cm), can be as hot as 100°F (38°C). The soil will not be completely sterilized but this heating promotes the beneficial organisms in the soil while killing or weakening the harmful ones.

Steps in Solarizing

1. Pick a time when the sun is hot. Locations that are warm all year round allow for solarizing at any time, but in cooler climates this process may need to be done in mid-summer. Depending on location, the temperature of the

soil can reach between 95 and 140°F (between 35 and 60°C).

2. The area of soil you are going to solarize should be free of plants.

3. Water the soil well. Moist soil conducts heat better than dry soil and makes soil-borne pests, weakened by the heat, more susceptible to beneficial organisms in the soil.

4. Cover the area with clear plastic, burying the edges to trap in the heat.

5. Leave the plastic sealed for four to six weeks, depending on geography. Warmer climates are ready sooner.

6. When the time is up, remove the plastic, allow the soil temperature to drop to normal, and plant.

Beating Weeds

Weeding is a garden chore that, much like washing the dishes, is never finished. It can be rewarding, however. It gets you outside in the sunshine. It's healthy exercise. You can eat many of the weeds you'll pull out. And you'll get a lot of satisfaction looking at a well-tended garden.

The definition of a weed is a plant that is growing in the wrong location. A rose bush growing in a corn patch is a weed. The plants most commonly called weeds tend to be a bit hardier and stronger, and often grow more quickly than other plants. Sometimes they are foreign medicinal herbs that were once valued but are now seen as invasive. Sometimes they are aggressive native species. Either way, they are basically disliked for being successful survivors. They don't need to be pampered. Most herbs do because they are not growing in their native habitats. Weeds compete with your desired herbs for space, food, water, light, and air. They also can carry diseases.

Don't put off the chore. I procrastinate with the best but I've learned it will make this job harder. It can be easy for the weeds to get the best of you if you don't stay on top of this job. That's exactly what happened to me with my first vegetable garden. I did so well for a while then ran low on time and let things go. Before I knew it, the weeds had taken over. Thankfully, most of my plants were big enough by then not to be bothered too much but the weeds were still competing for nutrients in the soil and that is never a good thing. Remove weeds weekly while their root systems are small. Large roots may disturb your herbs.

Weed after a rain. I'm not saying right after, while the soil is still muddy, but a day after while the soil is still soft but no longer wet. Those roots will pull more easily and more completely. If the area is going through a dry spell, water the day before you weed. Be very careful not to walk in a wet garden as it not only compacts the soil, but also increases the spread of disease.

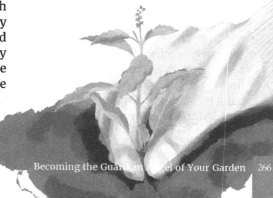

Pull the entire weed out, not just the leaves. Roots can't re-sprout if you pull the whole thing.

The old saying 'One year's seeding, seven years' weeding' documents the fact that most weed seeds live for many years in the soil. Do not allow weeds to grow big enough to go to seed and eventually you'll have fewer weeds to pull. Perennial weeds, especially, can make your gardening hard if you allow them to grow big.

Use all the help you can get. One way to reduce the number of weeds in a new garden is to use landscape cloth around your plants. The downside to landscape cloth is that it's synthetic and must be removed at least once a season to prevent it from breaking and contaminating the soil. It can also be expensive. Newspaper, at least five sheets thick, is as effective as black plastic and landscape cloth for smothering weeds. By spring, the newspaper will have degraded substantially, and will have rotted away completely by the end of the summer warm season. That makes this an environmentally friendly way to kill your weeds and keep something else out of a landfill. Cardboard also works – you finally have something to do with all those pizza boxes! Use mulch on top of the paper to keep it from blowing away and make it look more attractive. Mulch will also keep the soil moisture from evaporating while still allowing rain and air through.

Overwintering

After a hard frost has killed annuals and sent biennials and perennials dormant, and the wildlife has eaten what they will, clean up the garden. Pull dead annuals and second-year biennials. Refresh labels for things you've allowed to self-seed. It's too easy to forget exactly where they were located and then plant something else in that spot the following spring. Or, as I have done a couple times, plant the same thing and end up with an overabundance of one type of herb and not enough of another.

Tidy your garden by cutting to the ground the stems of herbs that die back. Dead stems can be whipped back and forth by winter winds that damage dormant roots and can carry disease into spring. Dead garden waste can be added to a compost pile. Avoid adding diseased plant matter to compost unless you have a 'hot pile' and can ensure that it gets hot enough to kill the disease agents. Even then, I wouldn't chance it because I would worry that the heat wouldn't kill off everything. Leave alone the herbs that resprout leaves from dormant stems or are evergreen.

If you live in an area where the soil doesn't usually freeze, a thick layer of mulch can protect plants from short dips in temperature. Apply the mulch when the soil is at normal temperature, to insulate it from the cold.

If you live where winters are snowy, mulch the garden after the ground is fully frozen to keep herbs dormant. Climate change has varied winter and spring temperatures making weather iffy. False springs, where the weather warms for a few weeks but then becomes icy again, have become normal in some areas, like mine. You want your herbs to stay dormant until the weather has stabilized and warmed for the season.

Beneficial Insects

When I was a kid, I had a reputation for playing with insects. A little weird, I know, but I loved the critters. I remember one time in particular when my mom and I went to visit her best friend and I was in their yard playing with wooly worms (fuzzy caterpillars that turn into tiger moths), and other random bugs. My mom's best friend told her that she had toys in the house that I could play with, but my mom replied that I was perfectly happy with my bugs; and she was absolutely right. And it hasn't changed. When I learned of all the ways in which insects benefit my beloved plants, that made me love them all the more. There are many kinds of beneficial insects. They differ from area to area. Familiarize yourself with both the larval and adult forms of local ones so you won't squash them. When you use a poison to kill what's eating your herb, unfortunately you also kill the beneficial insects. Before you resort to that, try waiting. Good bugs often trail bad bugs by about two weeks. But they do come, and come hungry! Below are listed a few that live in most areas.

Ladybugs, as they are called in North America, or ladybirds in Great Britain and other English speaking parts of the world, are small, red and black-spotted beetles that are a familiar sight in many gardens. They eat aphids, mites, scale insects and other soft-bodied, harmful bugs. Millions are raised each year for purchase. (Pro tip: when buying them for release in your garden, first put them in the fridge for 15 minutes to 'cool them down,' then release them at nighttime, so they don't just fly away. Instead they will crawl slowly onto the leaves and start munching on aphids!)

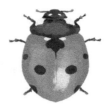

Lacewings are insects commonly found in North America and Europe. Another common name for them is stinkflies. Larvae are called 'aphid lions.' They eat aphids, mites, and other soft-bodied bugs. They are raised and sold as eggs since they are cannibalistic after they hatch.

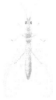

Assassin bugs have a long proboscis, which is a scientific term for 'nose,' with which they stab prey, inject saliva into its body, and suck the dissolved tissue out. They eat a great many pests and are generally regarded as a good bug, but be careful when handling one – it may give your finger a painful stab. The first time I saw one, I was amazed. I had no idea on earth what this crazy looking bug was, but its mouthpiece didn't look like something I wanted to mess with. After research, I was glad I hadn't tested my luck.

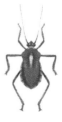

Fireflies are often called lightning bugs here in the south but they are not found in all regions. While adults eat pollen, nectar, other fireflies, or even nothing at all, the larvae are specialized predators that eat other insect larvae, snails, and slugs. There are no downsides to having them around as they don't bite, aren't poisonous/venomous, and don't carry diseases. Plus they make one heck of a light show at night. One of my favorite activities in summer is going out into the yard with the kids and catching fireflies as their lights slowly blink on and off (which they do to attract mates).

Populations of all types of pollinators are declining because of a combination of pollution, misuse of pesticides and other chemicals, disease and loss of habitat. You can, and absolutely should whenever possible, encourage pollinators by supporting practices that reduce pollution, using organic gardening methods, growing plants that feed pollinator babies (I love leaving some of my plants to go to flower just for the pollinators), supporting community gardens in cities, and providing other habitats such as bee houses and bat nesting boxes.

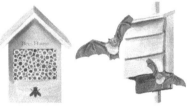

Pollinators

Honey bees are well known as pollinators but are not the only ones by far. Flowers were pollinated long before Europeans brought honey bees to North America. Honey bees are popular because they are manageable by humans. Thousands of hives are transported to crops each year. This actually causes some harm to indigenous pollinators. Bumblebees, mining bees, and many other kinds of bees, butterflies, and moths are some of our natural pollinators. Less popular pollinators include syrphid flies, blowflies, hoverflies, pollen wasps, ants, mosquitoes (only the female needs blood), and flower beetles. Certain birds and a few mammals – including bats and even humans – are also pollinators.

Spring Cleanup

Growing up, Nana taught me to keep mulch in place so that the soil would stay cold until the weather stabilized enough to prevent hard freezes. If the soil stays cold, your herbs will remain dormant. Global warming is changing our weather, though, and it's more up and down now. This causes plants to break dormancy before the winter is really over. New growth is much more vulnerable to the cold.

After the weather stabilizes, remove the mulch away from your herbs to allow the soil to warm. If your springs are as wet as mine, you may want to remove mulch completely as it holds water. Reapply after summer arrives to conserve water and suppress weeds.

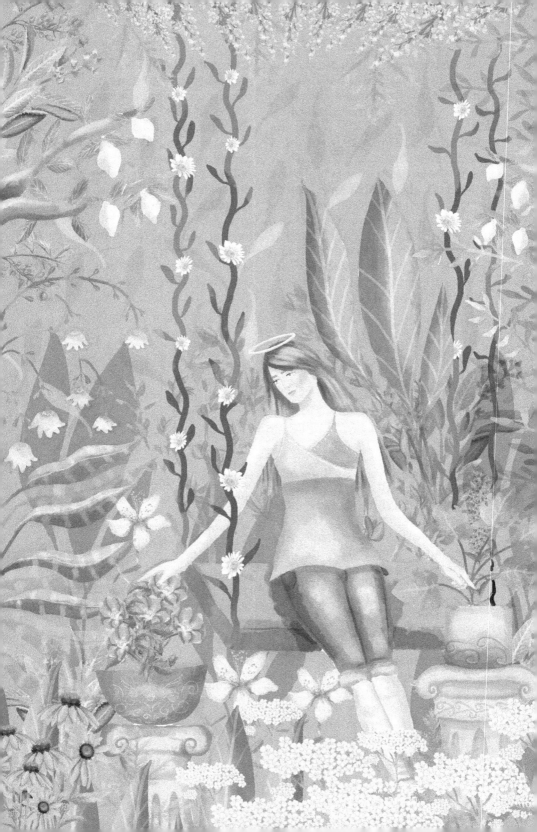

Conclusion

Congratulations, you've got all the way to the end; it's a bittersweet feeling, right? You feel great that it's finally done, but it was so much fun on the way and you want to keep learning about the herbal world …

But don't worry, if you haven't read 'The Art of Herbal Healing: Herbalism for Beginners,' that might be a great choice to go more deeply into how herbs actually work on YOUR body (see the link in the back of the book). Also, we are currently working on an herbs for children book, an herbs for moms (fertility and pregnancy) book, an herbs for pets book, hygiene with herbs (soaps, bathing, skincare) and more … Depending on when you read this, maybe ALL of these books will already have been released! Then you'd find them listed at the back of this book. We will keep you updated on our Facebook group.

Let's recap, in 'Grow Your Own Medicine' you've learned:

1. Many different reasons to grow your own culinary and medicinal herbs

2. The basics of gardening

3. The type of garden that is suitable for you, considering your living situation and hardiness zone

4. The details about 50+ herbs to know, grow and use

5. How to maintain your garden and keep the herbs safe from pests and diseases

From a health perspective, you know exactly how your herbs were raised and what substances they have been exposed to. Certain herbs may be cheaper to raise than to buy. I know that one of the biggest draws for me is the sheer satisfaction I feel at being able to walk out and pick my own herbs when I need them. And to know that what I harvest is the product of my own hand. I worked for this, and the pride I feel over my plants makes the produce taste so much better. Fresh items will always taste better and have more powerful medicinal effects.

There is a first small and very simple step I'd like you to take, to connect to Mother Nature and all her wonders. Start with two plants in pots. Any two plants you want. Start slowly with those plants; nurture them and see how things go. If you are anything like me, it won't take long for you to want more.

Also If you have found this book useful and valuable, consider gifting it to three people whom you think could really benefit from it. They could be your relatives, friends, colleagues, your favorite local small business owner, neighbor, or even someone you just met and wish to surprise. The crazy thing (well, maybe not that crazy, really) is that YOU can be the catalyst that helps your neighborhood begin to make beautiful, lush herb gardens that benefit not only you and your neighbors, but all of Mother Nature as well.

When you make a small, positive difference in another person's life, that same goodness is bound to return to you. Learning the beginning steps to grow a garden, through this book, could truly help someone's physical and psychological health, as gardening has done for me and so many others. And that person could receive this gift from you. Without you, they might never find out about the joy of gardening. Write down the names of the three people you believe would benefit from this knowledge and consider sending them a copy of this book:

1) _____

2) _____

3) _____

You made a great decision by choosing me as your guide, to help you take your first step towards a healthier and more fulfilling life. I look forward to seeing your successful herb garden on our Facebook group even if it's just one plant (although I'm willing to bet you can't stop at just one).

Welcome To YOUR Herb Garden!

A small favor

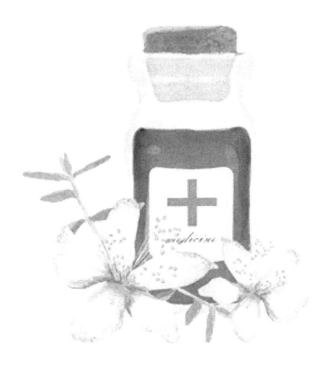

Did you learn a thing or two and enjoyed this book?
Please consider scanning the QR code below to leave a short review. These reviews cure my aching author heart.

It won't take longer than 30 seconds. It can be just a sentence or two. Thank you, it means alot to me.

References and further reading

Hardy, K., Buckley, S., Collins, M., Estalrrich, A., Brothwell, D., Copeland, L., Garcia-Tabernero, A., García-Vargas, S., Rasilla, M., Lalueza-Fox, C., Huguet, R., Bastir, M., Santamaría, D., Madella, M., Wilson, J., Fernandez-Cortes, A., & Rosas, A. (2012). Neanderthal medics? Evidence for food, cooking, and medicinal plants entrapped in dental calculus. Die Naturwissenschaften, 99, 617–26. DOI: 10.1007/s00114-012-0942-0.

Lassen, A. W., Frahm, E., & Wagensonner, K. IEds.). (2019). Ancient Mesopotamia speaks: Highlights of the Yale Babylonian collection. Yale Peabody Museum of Natural History. https://yalebooks.yale.edu/book/9781933789378/ancient-mesopotamia-speaks

Mahomoodally, M. F. (2013). Traditional medicines in Africa: an appraisal of ten potent African medicinal plants. Evidence-based Complementary and Alternative Medicine : eCAM, 617459. https://doi.org/10.1155/2013/617459

Gupta, J. L. (2013). Economic and Business Environment. Vision, 17(1), 83–85. https://doi.org/10.1177/0972262912469569

Scurlock, J., & Andersen, B. R. (2005). Diagnoses in Assyrian and Babylonian medicine: Ancient sources, translations, and modern medical analyses. University of Illinois Press. DOI: http://www.jstor.org/stable/10.5406/j.ctt2ttfm5

Fanouriou, E., Kalivas, D., Daferera, D., & Tarantillis, P. (2018). Hippocratic medicinal flora on the Greek Island of Kos: Spatial distribution, assessment of soil conditions, essential oil content and chemotype analysis. Journal of applied research on medicinal and aromatic plants, 9(1), 97–109. DOI: https://agris.fao.org/agris-search/search.do?recordID=US201900437568

Qitsualik, R. A. (2018). Of herbs and Inuit. Indian Country Today, Sept. 12.

Resources

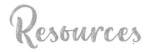

See the top herbalism books & other books by Ava

www.theherb.space/books

Your Tools Link

www.theherb.space/tools

FB groups join link

www.theherb.space/group

Ailments & Herb Properties Index

Ailments

Herb Properties

Recipes

Printed in the USA
CPSIA information can be obtained
at www.ICGtesting.com
LVHW021702130124
768548LV00157B/5576